OTHER VOLUMES IN
EXERCISES IN DIAGNOSTIC RADIOLOGY

Published

Forthcoming

EXERCISES IN DIAGNOSTIC RADIOLOGY

6

NUCLEAR RADIOLOGY

A. EVERETTE JAMES, Jr., Sc.M., M.D.

Associate Professor of Radiology and
Director, Radiological Research,
Department of Radiology, The Johns Hopkins
Hospital, Baltimore, Maryland

LUCY FRANK SQUIRE, M.D.

Professor of Radiology, Downstate
Medical Center, Brooklyn, New York;
Consultant in Radiology, Massachusetts General
Hospital, Boston, Massachusetts

W. B. SAUNDERS COMPANY • PHILADELPHIA • LONDON • TORONTO

W. B. Saunders Company: West Washington Square
Philadelphia, Pa. 19105

12 Dyott Street
London, WC1A 1DB

833 Oxford Street
Toronto, Ontario M8Z 5T9, Canada

Exercises in Diagnostic Radiology – Volume 6   Nuclear Radiology   ISBN 0-7216-5103-8

Print No.:   9   8   7   6   5   4   3   2

PREFACE

The purpose of this text is to introduce the reader to certain aspects of a new specialty, nuclear medicine. Only the imaging characteristics and their complementary nature to the radiograph will be emphasized. This does not mean that we fail to appreciate the great value of the in vitro tests or the physiological and quantitative data derived by this safe, simple and innocuous investigative technique, but the purpose of *The Exercises* is to focus upon abnormal image patterns.

Disease processes are manifestations of altered physiology. Recognizable structural changes are useful because they offer the informed observer clues to the abnormality of function that exists. In radiology it soon became evident that often a static image did not provide the continuum of observation necessary to arrive at an accurate diagnosis. As a result, fluoroscopic, contrast and angiographic techniques were developed which allowed sequential analysis of specific organ and body functions. Diagnostic nuclear medicine employs minute amounts of radioactivity to trace physiological processes and to record structural information. Although the images obtained, even with the present sophisticated devices, do not possess the structural definition of their radiographic counterparts, they do contain clinically useful physiological data because of the manner in which the radioactivity is acquired, accumulated and localized in the area of interest.

In this volume we shall continually call the reader's attention to this type of information and ask him to think "physiologically with an anatomical bias." He should carefully analyze the structural information present on the radiograph and scan, while remembering the physiological principle employed to localize the radioactivity to that particular organ, compartment or area.

We have followed a familiar pattern in dividing the considerations of this text according to organ systems. In the introduction to each chapter there will be a brief statement regarding the principles involved to achieve that particular image. For a survey of the basic principles employed in nuclear medicine, the reader is referred to several general texts on the subject. For the uninitiated we recommend *Clinical Nuclear Medicine* by Maynard and the multi-volume *Atlas of Nuclear Medicine* by DeLand and Wagner. Those interested in a detailed consideration of all aspects of the specialty might attempt Wagner's *Principles of Nuclear Medicine* or Blahd's *Nuclear Medicine*. These reference texts consider in much greater detail the methods employed to achieve the images shown in these exercises. Of course, this book is in no way a substitute for those just mentioned, but is an exercise in image perception and correlation, emphasizing the complementary approach of nuclear medicine and radiology.

ACKNOWLEDGMENTS

Any text requires the assistance of many persons who contribute in various ways, including some through moral support and others by negative input to keep the authors honest. To the Johns Hopkins medical students who reviewed the text "in the rough" and pointed out the areas that were poorly explained, did not teach them anything or were insufficiently emphasized, we owe a profound "thanks." Sampling our intended audience proved to be a tremendous learning experience for us. The Fellows in the Division of Nuclear Medicine at Johns Hopkins read the manuscript in their areas of particular interest and offered many useful suggestions; they also were most helpful in collecting the cases. Particular thanks go to Drs. Henry Wagner, Harold DeBlanc, Pablo Dibos, David Moses, Fred Lomas, Paul Dugal, Peter Kirchner, Frank DeLand, Peter J. Hurley, Hadwig Wesselhoeft, David C. Moses, and Ken McKusik for specific patients. Dr. Fred Jenner Hodges, III, was especially gracious in helping us to select the cases reviewed in the section, Brain and Cerebrospinal Fluid. Dr. Wagner was the source of many of the principles and "take home messages" that have proved diagnostically sound.

Three "experts" reviewed the manuscripts for mistakes. Paul B. Hoffer, Robert I. White and Charles E. Jordan performed this task with interest, diligence and compassion. Miss Wendy North assisted in many ways as she aided in collecting cases and advised with the manuscript format. Drs. Martin W. Donner, Henry N. Wagner, Jr., and Russell H. Morgan made available the resources of the Departments of Radiology and Radiological Sciences. Henri Hessels and Willie Ragsdale did the photography and Mrs. David Levin, the typing. The Department of Art as Applied to Medicine is responsible for many of the drawings.

We are grateful to those persons who have allowed their illustrations to be reproduced herein.

The W. B. Saunders Company was most cooperative, patient and understanding. Jack Hanley kept encouraging us to completion.

A. EVERETTE JAMES, JR., Sc.M., M.D.

LUCY F. SQUIRE, M.D.

CONTENTS

CHAPTER I

LUNG

LUNG SCANNING

Evaluation of respiratory disease using radiopharmaceuticals generally depends upon assessment of pulmonary circulation and evaluation of ventilatory function. The most common clinical situation in which the lung scan has been utilized is in the detection of pulmonary emboli. However, many other important clinical uses are being found for this diagnostic study.

Perfusion lung scans depend upon the particle distribution of radioactively labeled substances (usually macroaggregates or microspheres of albumin) which reflect the distribution of pulmonary arterial blood flow. The capillaries in the lung act as filters and entrap particles that are larger than 7 to 8 microns in diameter. Therefore, after intravenous injection, labeled particles larger than the mean diameter of the capillaries of the lung will become lodged for a limited period of time in the capillary bed (drawing, Figure 1 A). The distribution of radioactivity reflects regional pulmonary arterial blood flow. Areas of diminished perfusion will be seen as areas of decreased radioactivity.

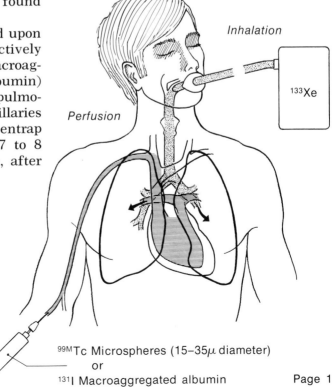

Inhalation

^{133}Xe

Perfusion

Figure 1 A. *Lung imaging.*

^{99M}Tc Microspheres (15–35μ diameter)
or
^{131}I Macroaggregated albumin

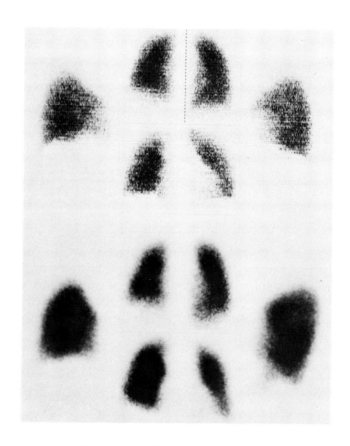

Figure 1 B. *Normal rectilinear perfusion lung scan (above) and camera perfusion lung scan (below). (From DeLand, F. H., and Wagner, H. N.:* Atlas of Nuclear Medicine, Vol. 2, *1970.)*

The normal distribution of radioactivity is uniform throughout both lung fields when the patient is injected intravenously with the labeled particles while in the supine position. (Figures 1 B and 3). If the patient is injected while erect or sitting upright, there will be generalized diminished radioactivity in the upper lung fields. This reflects the fact that normally, in the vertical position, pulmonary arterial blood flow to the upper lobes of the lung is less than to the lower.

Any abnormality which causes a localized decrease in pulmonary blood flow will be seen as a discrete area of diminished radioactivity. Lesions that are primary in the pulmonary arterial bed cannot be separated from those within the lung parenchyma which secondarily affect pulmonary blood flow. Both will be reflected as decreased areas of radioactivity. Therefore, it is essential that perfusion lung scans be interpreted concomitantly with a good quality chest radiograph obtained at the time of the lung scan.

Ventilatory function of the lung can be assessed by inhalation of a radioactive gas (drawing, Figure 1 A), intravenous injection of a radioactive substance which diffuses out of the pulmonary vascular system and into the alveoli, or by inhalation of radioactively labeled submicron-sized particles. The distribution of radioactivity at various time intervals during the study will provide information about the multiple parameters of ventilatory function. The various phases have been referred to as the "wash-in," equilibrium and "wash-out" phases of the ventilatory cycle (Figure 2).

Various disease states are reflected by abnormalities in the different phases of the ventilatory cycle. For example, pulmonary embolism will show a perfusion abnormality initially, but no abnormality within the ventilatory portion of the inhalation study. Therefore, the ventilatory or inhalation scans of the lung have been utilized to differentiate acute pulmonary embolism from chronic obstructive lung disease. Parenchymal lung disease often shows the normal "wash-in" and equilibrium phase of the ventilatory cycle, but a delay in the "wash-out" phase. This delay is manifest as continued concentration of the radiopharmaceutical in a particular region of the lung. Obstructive lesions of the major bronchi will show abnormalities throughout all phases of the inhalation study.

Remember, by the inhalation method, the radiopharmaceutical is delivered to the terminal bronchi and alveoli, depending upon whether or not the bronchial lumen is patent. With many forms of parenchymal lung disease the bronchial lumen will allow the radiopharmaceutical to enter distal structures on inspiration. When large bronchi are obstructed, no radiopharmaceutical will pass through the lumen and no radioactivity appear distally.

The value of these studies in assessing regional pulmonary function has been realized only partially.

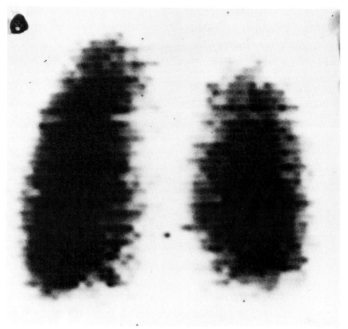

Figure 2 A. Normal xenon study (wash in phase).

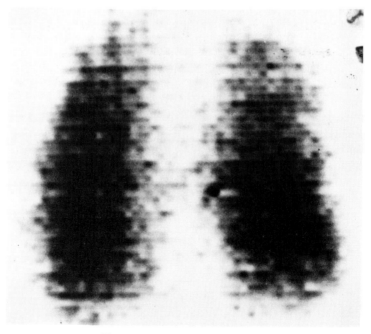

Figure 2 B. Normal xenon study (equilibrium phase).

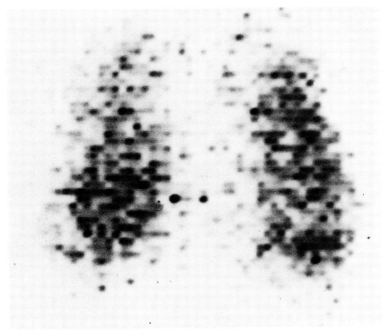

Figure 2 C. Normal xenon study (washout phase, 4 seconds after breathing room air).

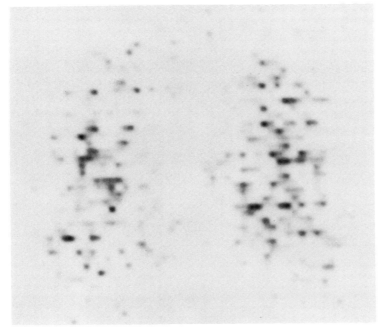

Figure 2 D. Normal xenon study (washout phase, 16 seconds after breathing room air).

INTERPRETATION OF
THE LUNG SCAN

Following the intravenous injection of an appropriate radiopharmaceutical, the patient is oriented in front of a detection crystal (usually thallium-activated sodium iodide) to obtain the various views of the perfusion lung scan. For the anterior view (Figure 3 A) the anterior chest wall is closer to the detection crystal than the posterior structures in the chest. When the lateral views are obtained, the patient is usually lying on his side (Figure 3 C and D), and the side which is being imaged is closest to the imaging device. When the rectilinear scanner is employed as the imaging device, the patient is usually imaged while supine. The patient's lung scan may be obtained in the upright position when the scintillation camera is utilized.

When the patient is injected in the supine position, the distribution of radioactivity on the perfusion lung scan should be homogeneous (drawing, Figure 3 E). However, there is often a slight generalized decrease of radioactivity in the upper lung fields because of less lung volume in the apices. The superior mediastinum is seen as a wide linear band of diminished radioactivity on the anterior view (Figure 3 A). The entire mediastinum is visualized in the same manner on the posterior view (Figure 3 B). The cardiac silhouette is best seen on the anterior view. The left ventricle is noted as an area of diminished activity oriented laterally and somewhat obliquely downward to the left (Figure 3 A and E). Hilar structures are sometimes seen as negative areas of radioactivity adjacent to the mediastinum. If these are well delineated, one should suspect enlargement of the pulmonary artery or lymph nodes. Inferiorly at the diaphragmatic margin there may be linear areas of diminished activity or irregular activity resulting from respiratory motion during the examination. An upward curvature of the basilar radioactivity is often present in obese patients owing to hypoventilation and hypoperfusion of the lower lung fields. This hypoperfusion is present as a physiological variant in obese patients and must be distinguished from pleural disease or pleural effusion, which can give a similar appearance.

There is considerable difference in the right and left lateral views. On the left lateral (Figure 3 D), anteriorly, a diminished area of radioactivity which corresponds to the position of the heart is present. This may also be seen in the right lateral view (Figure 3 C) in cardiac enlargement, but is not nearly so distinct or prominent in the normal patient.

On the posterior view (Figure 3 B) the mediastinum appears as a band of diminished activity and the cardiac silhouette is not so well delineated as on the anterior view. There is generalized and homogeneous radioactivity throughout the lung fields. The normal decrease in radioactivity in the apical region is not so prominent as on the anterior view. Thinking anatomically, can you reason why this should be? Would it be true in a patient with kyphosis?

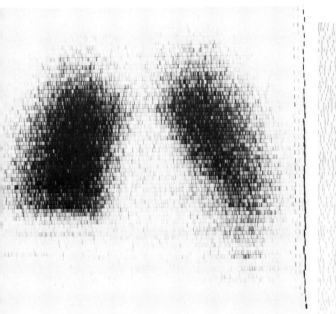

Figure 3 A. *Anterior.*

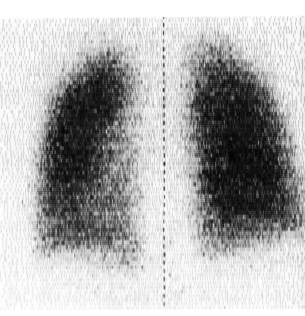

Figure 3 B. *Posterior.*

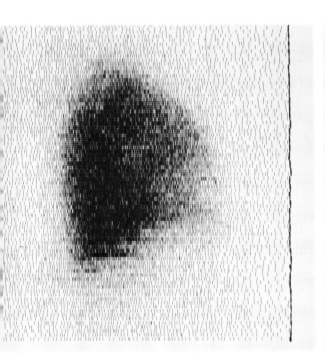

Figure 3 C. *Right lateral.*

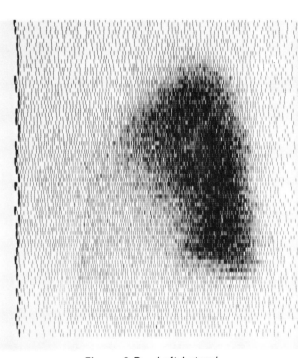

Figure 3 D. *Left Lateral.*

(Figure 3 A, B, C & D from DeLand, F. H., and Wagner, H. N.: Atlas of Nuclear Medicine, *Volume 2, 1970.)*

When the average chest is viewed in profile, the dorsal surface is relatively flat compared to the ventral. Because the amount of radioactivity reaching the detection crystal and recorded on the image depends upon the attenuation of the radioactivity before it reaches the face of the crystal, this anatomical difference affects the appearance of the anterior and posterior scans. Anteriorly the slope of the chest, as well as the decreased lung volume in the apices, results in less radioactivity being recorded superiorly by the imaging system than in the lower lung fields. The plane of best resolution of the collimator may be located close to the chest wall anteriorly but within the lung (or the field containing radioactivity) posteriorly. In a patient with kyphosis, both the anterior and posterior views might show diminished activity in the upper lung zones.

Oblique views of the lung scan can be obtained. The normal expected anatomy is somewhat distorted and occasionally difficult to interpret. The major utility of oblique views has been to aid in the decision of whether or not perfusion defects correspond to lung segments. This decision is of great clinical importance because, in general, perfusion defects caused by pulmonary emboli are segmental or subsegmental. Those defects caused by chronic lung disease are focal and usually not segmental (Figure 3 F), whereas perfusion defects characteristic of interstitial pulmonary edema are neither focal nor segmental (Figure 3 G). This might be expected if you consider that pulmonary embolism is a disease primarily involving the vessel lumen and that the other diseases affect the vessel only secondarily.

The various views of the lung scan should always be analyzed with the concomitant chest radiographs. They should be viewed simultaneously but oriented in some logical sequence. For purposes of case presentation we have chosen only the most illustrative views and have oriented them to correspond with the usual manner in which one views the related chest radiograph.

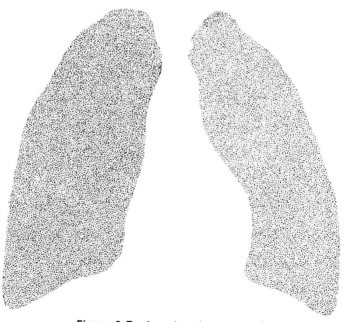

Figure 3 E. *Anterior view: normal.*

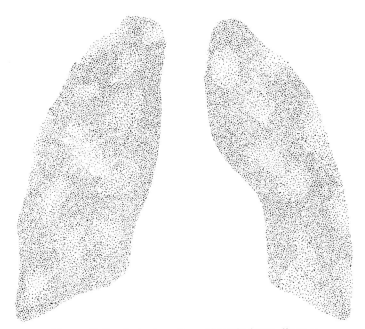

Figure 3 F. *Anterior view: chronic lung disease.*

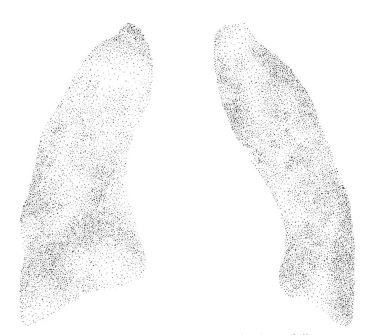

Figure 3 G. *Anterior view: congestive heart failure.*

PROBLEM

Sidney Sidewinder, 63, sustained a blow to his left side while attending a post-holiday sale in a fashionable women's lingerie shoppe. After several weeks of continued chest pain on the left side he was brought to the emergency room because of hemoptysis.

A perfusion lung scan was obtained after an intravenous radiopharmaceutical injection (Figure 4). This posterior view was made with the patient supine. Is the radioactivity uniform through both lungs? How would you characterize the abnormalities?

Now that you have decided whether or not perfusion defects are present and where they are, analyze the chest radiograph (Figure 5). Does the bilateral hilar calcification suggest any broad disease category? Did you overlook the more obvious abnormality in the left upper chest? Remember that any systematic approach to analysis of a chest radiograph includes the osseous structures as well as the lung parenchyma.

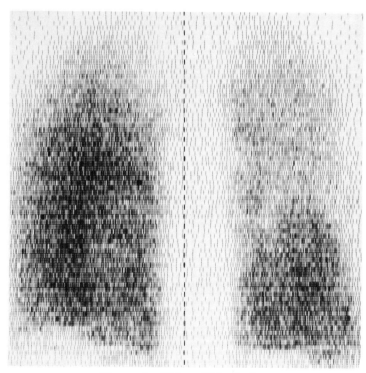

Figure 4. *Sidney Sidewinder.*

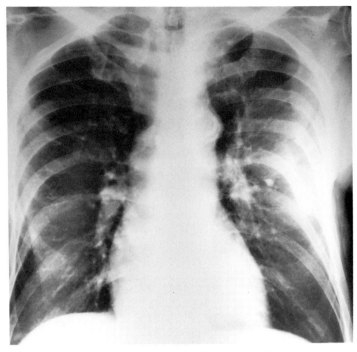

Figure 5. *Mr. Sidewinder's chest radiograph.*

ANSWER: The posterior lung scan shows minimal diminished radioactivity in the right upper lobe medially and a large defect involving the entire left upper lung field.

On the chest radiograph an explanation for the large left perfusion defect is seen. The left posterior 5th, 6th and 7th ribs have been fractured. This is not acute, as callus formation is present.

The small perfusion defect in the right upper lung field is probably a chronic change due to granulomatous disease. More important is the large area of decreased perfusion in the left upper lobe. This is a secondary effect from the trauma to the ribs.

PEARL: Similar perfusion defects may occur without rib fractures in closed chest trauma. Splinting of one side of the chest due to pain can result in areas of atelectasis and hypoperfusion, causing defects on the lung scan.

TEACHING POINT: Perfusion defects may be caused by a number of physio-

logical processes that alter regional pulmonary blood flow: trauma, splinting and postoperative atelectasis are examples of these. The changes in the right lung were attributed to chronic granulomatous disease. No segmental perfusion defects characteristic of pulmonary embolism were seen.

PROBLEM
Barry Hurry, 32, missed the lingerie sale completely because of an automobile accident. However, he also received a severe injury to his left side and entered the emergency room at the hospital in extreme respiratory distress. Soft tissue trauma to his left chest was apparent on physical examination. No rib fractures were detected and no pneumothorax was seen on the admission chest radiograph. After several hours in the hospital he became extremely short of breath. Pulmonary thromboembolism was considered and a lung scan was obtained (Figure 6).

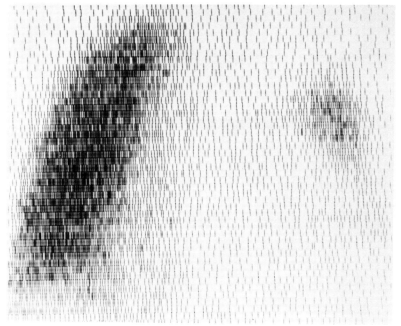

Figure 6. Barry Hurry.

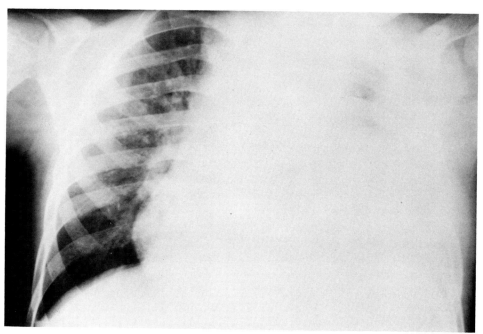

Figure 7. Barry's supine chest radiograph.

This anterior view is definitely abnormal, and one might consider a massive pulmonary embolus on his left. Thinking about the expected radiographic signs of an acute pulmonary embolus, does the chest radiograph (Figure 7) suggest that diagnosis?

ANSWER: On the anterior view minimal irregularity of radioactivity distribution is present on the right side, but almost no perfusion is present on the left. The concomitant chest radiograph reveals a possible cause for the perfusion defect.

The left hemithorax is generally dense, with only a small amount of normal lung present in the left upper lobe. With closed chest trauma, fluid density may appear in the lung as a result of parenchymal contusion, rupture of a vessel or alveolar pulmonary edema resulting from rapid change in intrathoracic pressure at impact. Interstitial pulmonary edema is present on the right side, presumably due to a shift of blood flow from the left side.

TEACHING POINT: The irregular "spotty" perfusion on the right is commonly seen with pulmonary edema. A hemothorax is present on the left. The presence of fluid around the pulmonary vessels greatly increases resistance to flow and prevents delivery of the radiopharmaceutical to the capillaries in that area.

Take Home Message: Stay away from post-holiday sales? No. Chest trauma can lead to perfusion defects by a variety of mechanisms. There may be profound physiological effects upon the pulmonary blood flow without parenchymal changes on the chest radiograph.

PROBLEM

Clarence "Red" Raider, 73, had long-standing tuberculosis and was being evaluated for chest surgery. Should his entire left lung be removed? Is there any viable lung on the left? What is the functional status of the right lung? Can it support respiratory function?

We have chosen only a single anterior view of the perfusion lung scan (Figure 8) to compare with the chest radiograph (Figure 9).

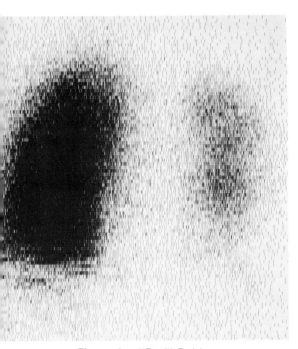

Figure 8. *"Red" Raider.*

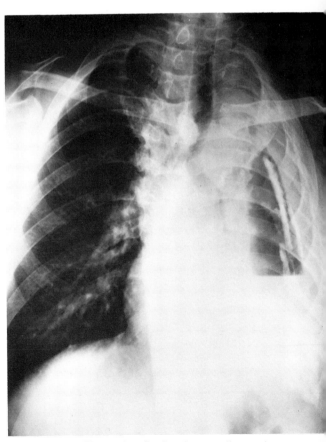

Figure 9. *Red's chest radiograph.*

INTERPRETATION: The anterior lung scan shows normal perfusion in the right lung and better than anticipated perfusion in the left lung. On the chest radiograph, pleural thickening, calcification, paratracheal calcification and an air-fluid level in the pleural space are present. These are characteristic of chronic granulomatous disease with an effusion.

PRACTICAL IMPORTANCE: Prior to removal of a lung, a lobe or any part thereof, it is important to know how much that part contributes to the patient's total lung function. To do this you must have some method of representing regional lung function in the area of disease as well as in the "normal" lung. The lung scan (perfusion + inhalation) is a simple procedure to acquire the data necessary for this assessment.

Use of lung imaging has had its greatest impetus from the clinical problem of detection of pulmonary emboli. Clinical manifestations of tachycardia, shortness of breath, chest pain and hemoptysis may have other etiologies. Serum enzyme measurements and electrocardiographic signs are often nonspecific and may even be normal. Unfortunately the many radiographic abnormalities that have been considered characteristic for pulmonary embolism in the past have not proved as reliable as initially expected. Pleural effusion, atelectasis and elevation of the diaphragm, dilatation of the central pulmonary artery segment, and absence of peripheral vessels are all radiographic manifestations associated with pulmonary embolism. None are specific; some are seen only rarely in our experience.

Most often in acute pulmonary embolism you will be faced with an abnormal perfusion lung scan with segmental perfusion defects and a chest radiograph that does not have abnormalities that explain the lung scan findings. You will often have obtained a chest radiograph on a patient suspected of having pulmonary embolism before considering a lung scan as a further diagnostic test. There may be abnormalities such as effusion, parenchymal densities or consolidation present on the chest radiograph that predictably will cause perfusion defects. In this situation is a lung scan helpful? Why?

Yes, it is helpful in that there are often segmental perfusion defects in areas where the chest radiograph is normal. As a screening device the lung scan is an extremely sensitive test for pulmonary emboli; it is not as *specific* as we would like. Conversely, the pulmonary angiogram is a very specific test for pulmonary embolism; it is not as *sensitive* as we would like. Small emboli lodging in vessels less than 2 mm. in diameter may cause perfusion defects involving several centimeters of lung in the periphery and yet not be detected by the pulmonary angiogram. You can imagine that the lung scan can be used profitably by the angiographer as a "road map" to select the vessel in which he would like to inject contrast. Radiographic magnification techniques to optimize visualization of these small peripheral vessels is also helpful.

Pulmonary emboli are considered to be the most likely diagnosis if segmental defects are present or if there is a rapidly changing pattern of perfusion defects on serial lung scans.

Angiographic signs for pulmonary emboli fall into two general categories which you could predict from your knowledge of anatomy and physiology:

A. Specific (primary signs)
  1. Filling defects in the contrast (caused by the emboli)
  2. Abrupt "cut-off" of a vessel filled with contrast
B. Nonspecific (secondary signs)
  1. Delayed contrast flow into the lung area supplied by that pulmonary artery, and late venous filling in the corresponding region
  2. Tapering of pulmonary vessels in a specific region

Now, with these "pearls" fresh in our minds, let's consider a series of patients clinically suspected for various reasons of having pulmonary emboli.

PROBLEM

Percival Epsom, 39, entered the hospital with severe abdominal pain, an elevated serum amylase and a clinical diagnosis of pancreatitis. Five days later he turned over in bed, experienced a sudden chest pain and was found to be cyanotic. With appropriate therapy his symptoms diminished and he had a lung scan several hours later (Figure 10). His chest radiograph at this time was entirely normal.

With a normal chest radiograph would you have predicted a perfusion lung scan of this bizarre nature? Would you then predict that this is primarily an intravascular or a parenchymal disorder?

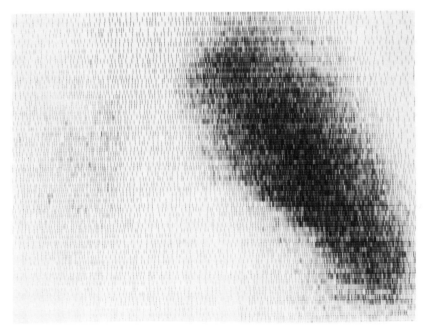

Figure 10. *Percival Epsom.*

INTERPRETATION: The anterior view perfusion lung scan shows almost total absence of perfusion on the right. *This striking finding may occur in pulmonary embolism, with lung cancer, following chest trauma, with pneumonia and after surgical palliation of certain congenital heart defects.* He had had no antecedent history and his chest radiograph was normal. This probably eliminates chest trauma, pneumonia and surgical palliation as reasonable possibilities. A central neoplasm in the right hilar region will usually be detected by a good quality chest radiograph.

This patient is very ill and we must provide him with immediate definitive therapy. Will pulmonary angiography establish the diagnosis? Given this large a perfusion defect, you would predict that the patient has a large pulmonary embolus lodged in the right pulmonary artery. We ought to be able to delineate this quite clearly on the pulmonary angiogram.

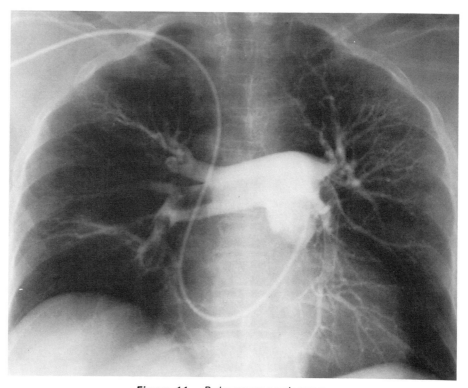

Figure 11. *Pulmonary angiogram.*

ANSWER: The pulmonary angiogram (Figure 11) reveals a large intravascular defect in the contrast in the main pulmonary artery and extending to the right side, diagnostic of pulmonary embolus. The left lower lobe embolus does not appear to obstruct blood flow to that lobe sufficient to cause a recognizable perfusion defect.

PROBLEM

Tiny Edgar Chance, 58, had a recent episode of chest pain without hemoptysis or shortness of breath. WBC 8000, respirations 20, pulse 88. His electrocardiogram showed left ventricular enlargement. Serum enzyme studies have not returned from the laboratory. This chest radiograph (Figure 12) and perfusion lung scan (posterior and both lateral views) (Figure 13 A, B and C) were obtained. Are radiographic changes present to explain the perfusion defects on the lung scan? Do the perfusion defects appear segmental in nature on the combination of posterior and lateral views?

Before showing you the *angiogram* performed on the same day as the initial lung scan, let's analyze the lung scan obtained two days later (Figure 14 A, B and C). Would you expect this sequence of changes in chronic lung disease?

INTERPRETATION: The chest radiograph demonstrates cardiomegaly, which appears mainly left ventricular in contour. Centrally the pulmonary arteries are prominent, but no marked decrease in pulmonary vessels peripherally is present. No parenchymal densities, pleural effusion or changes of chronic lung disease are detected.

The posterior and lateral views of the initial lung scan show multiple perfusion defects, many of which are segmental or subsegmental in distribution. On the right lateral, the posterior segment of the upper lobe and lateral and posterior basilar segments of the right lower lobe are easily identified. Other perfusion defects in the left lung are not quite so easily placed in a segmental distribution. Only the lateral basilar segmental defect in the right lower lobe (Figure 14 B) persists on the third scan, along with scattered areas of irregular distribution of radioactivity.

These serial changes add to our confidence in the diagnosis, but remember you had to begin proper treatment at the time of the *first* lung scan. So, you had to select the diagnostic study that would give a specific answer—and you decided upon a pulmonary angiogram.

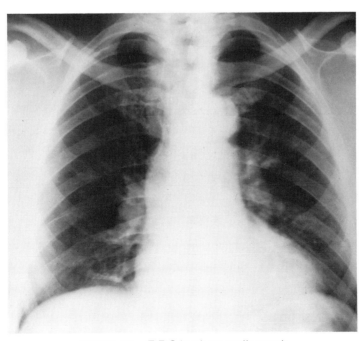

Figure 12. *T.E.C.'s chest radiograph.*

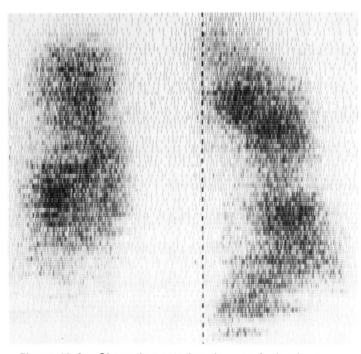

Figure 13 A. *Chance's posterior view, perfusion lung scan.*

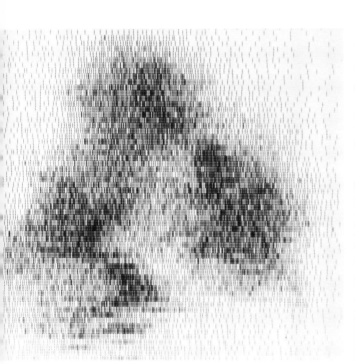

Figure 13 B. *Right lateral view.*

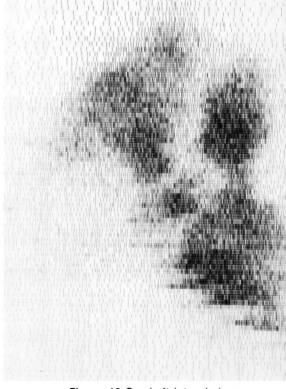

Figure 13 C. *Left lateral view.*

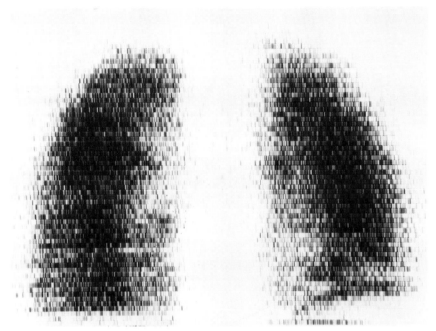

Figure 14 A. *Chance's posterior lung scan (two days later).*

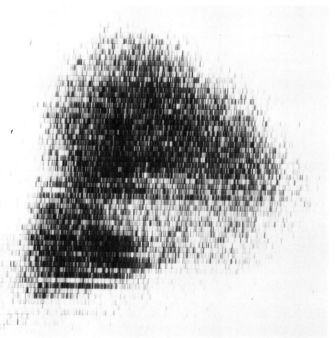

Figure 14 B. *Right lateral view (two days later).*

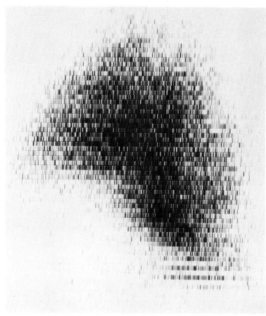

Figure 14 C. *Left lateral view (two days later).*

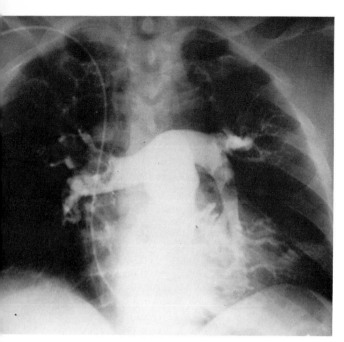

Figure 15 A. *T.E.C.'s pulmonary angiogram (arterial phase).*

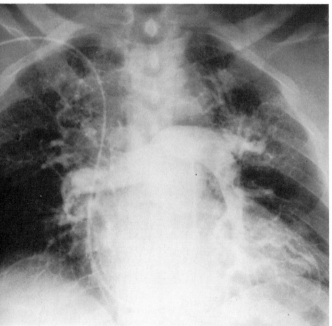

Figure 15 B. *Chance's angiogram (late arterial phase).*

Figure 15 C. *Chance's angiogram (selective study, left pulmonary artery).*

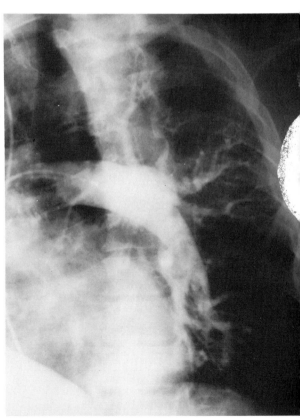

ANSWER: With injection of contrast, in the early phase of the angiogram (Figure 15 A), multiple intravascular filling defects are present in the right main pulmonary artery and its branches to the right upper and lower lobes as well as in the left lower lobe branch of the pulmonary artery. The later phase (Figure 15 B) shows delayed flow of contrast to these areas and a relatively avascular left upper lobe. Selective left main pulmonary artery injection (Figure 15 C) more clearly delineates the intravascular filling defects in the left pulmonary artery and demonstrates defects in the contrast not detected on the routine views.

Diagnosis: Pulmonary embolism with subsequent lysis due to urokinase infusion.

TEACHING POINT: Multiple segmental defects, not explained by abnormalities on the chest radiograph, that change with serial scans are almost certainly pulmonary emboli. However, therapy such as urokinase infusion can alter the perfusion pattern.

PROBLEM

Mary Gee, 38, has had episodic "spells" of wheezing and shortness of breath over the past several years. There has been no associated hemoptysis or fever. The chest radiograph was normal except for cardiomegaly. A lung scan (Figure 16 *A* and *B*) was performed because of the possibility of multiple recurrent pulmonary emboli. Besides the cardiomegaly you already knew she had, is this scan abnormal? Are the perfusion defects segmental or nonsegmental?

INTERPRETATION: Multiple small perfusion defects are present on the anterior and posterior view of the perfusion lung scan. These are probably subsegmental in distribution. Several are large enough to be considered segmental. Did we fail to mention that the patient was wheezing during the study?

Continued on following page.

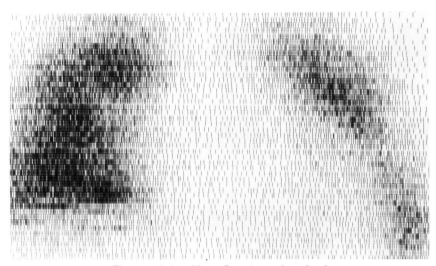

Figure 16 A. *Mary Gee (anterior view).*

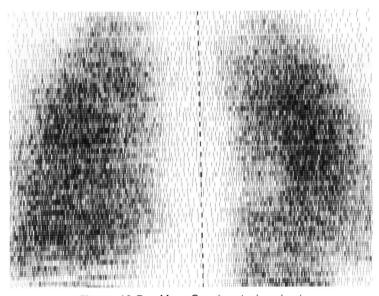

Figure 16 B. *Mary Gee (posterior view).*

Miss Gee's routine laboratory data were entirely normal. There was little enthusiasm for the diagnosis of pulmonary embolism in this patient, but the multiple defects on the lung scan had to be taken seriously and a pulmonary angiogram was obtained (Figure 17).

INTERPRETATION: A pulmonary angiogram performed several hours after the initial lung scan is normal.

CLUE: Although by far the most common cause of segmental perfusion defects is pulmonary emboli, patients will manifest this type of abnormality during asthmatic attacks.

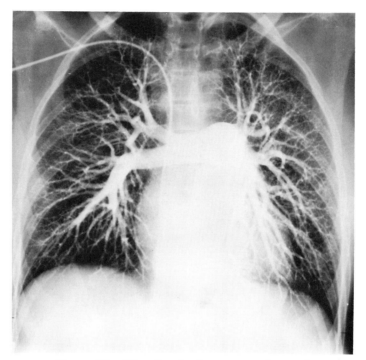

Figure 17. Miss Gee (pulmonary angiogram).

ANSWER: A repeat lung scan (Figure 18 *A* and *B*) following therapy for asthma and at a time when the patient was not wheezing shows cardiomegaly and a single perfusion defect on the right. The patient's subsequent serum enzyme determinations were normal. She was considered to have had an acute asthmatic episode.

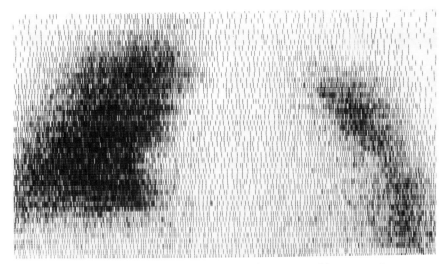

Figure 18 A. Miss Gee (anterior view, second lung scan).

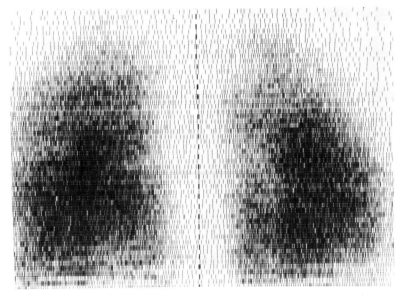

Figure 18 B. Miss Gee (posterior view, second lung scan).

TEACHING POINT: If a patient is wheezing at the time of the lung scan we often defer the study and reschedule after appropriate therapy. The pathophysiological changes that occur during an acute asthmatic attack will cause segmental perfusion defects.

PROBLEM

William Wheeze, 61, suffered an episode of severe substernal crushing chest pain one day before his lung scan. After routine laboratory studies proved uninformative, this study (Figure 19) was performed because of persistent dyspnea. A corresponding detail of his chest radiograph is shown in Figure 20.

Do you think that the distribution of radioactivity is homogeneous? Are the defects focal or nonfocal in nature? Might they even be described as generalized?

The selected view of the right lung has been chosen for you to particularly note the air-vessel wall interface (Figure 20). Is this clearly delineated? What are some of the common causes of blurring of this margin?

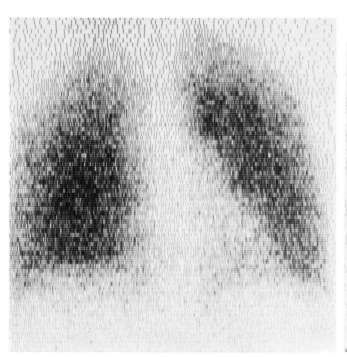

Figure 19 A. William Wheeze.

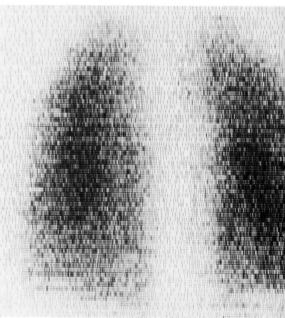

Figure 19 B. William Wheeze (posterior view

INTERPRETATION: There is respiratory motion present on the posterior lung scan and generalized irregular distribution of radioactivity on the anterior and posterior views. The patient was in respiratory distress during the study. Minimal cardiomegaly is seen on the anterior scan as well as multiple small nonsegmental perfusion defects.

CLUE: Remember that the distribution of the labeled microspheres depends upon the integrity of pulmonary vasculature from the main pulmonary artery to the capillary bed. If small vessels have increased resistance, the radiopharmaceutical will not be delivered to the area supplied by those vessels. The selected radiographic view during the patient's episode (Figure 20) should offer one explanation for the scan pattern.

The interface between the air in the lung parenchyma and the vessel wall is indistinct. Septal (Kerley B) lines are present. Probably the commonest cause of this radiographic appearance is interstitial pulmonary edema. Heart failure leading to pulmonary edema commonly follows myocardial infarction, which would explain the sudden onset of chest pain.

This patient does, indeed, have interstitial pulmonary edema resulting from an acute myocardial infarction.

TEACHING POINT: Left ventricular failure results in perivascular "cuffing" of small pulmonary vessels. This elevates interstitial pressure around the vessel and increases resistance to flow in the vessel. Many small pulmonary vessels collapse, preventing delivery of the radiopharmaceutical peripherally in the lung from an intravenous injection. Thus, the distribution of radioactivity will be irregular, and multiple nonfocal nonsegmental perfusion defects will be seen on the lung scan.

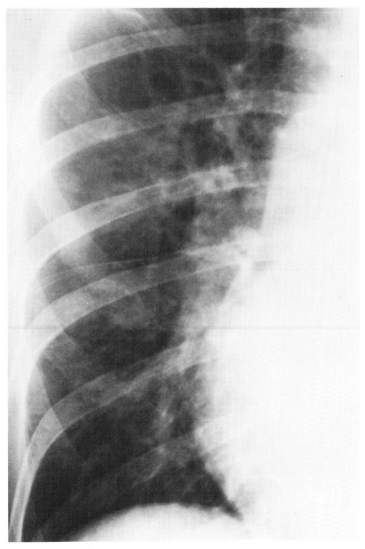

Figure 20. William Wheeze.

PROBLEM

Felicity Wolkstone, 48, also had an acute myocardial infarction. She was cyanotic when seen in the emergency room, where this chest radiograph was obtained (Figure 21).

Because of the marked respiratory difficulty and abnormal chest radiograph, she also had a perfusion lung scan (Figure 22). How would you describe the densities on the chest radiograph? Are these defects primarily alveolar or interstitial? Would you have predicted that the radiographic densities (which you doubtless recognized as alveolar pulmonary edema) would cause perfusion defects and, if so, would they be focal or nonfocal?

Focal perfusion defects are present on the posterior view. Do these defects correspond in position and location to the densities present on the chest radiograph?

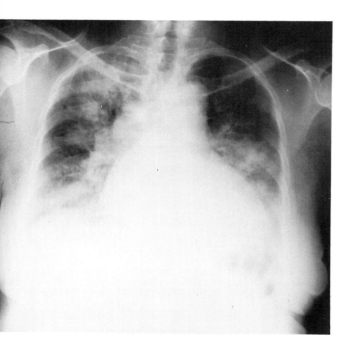

Figure 21. Miss Wolkstone.

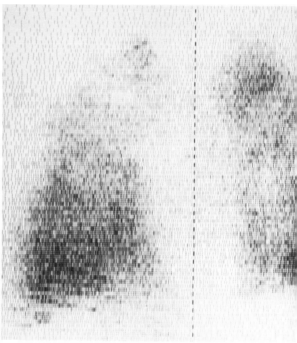

Figure 22. Felicity Wolkstone (posterior view, perfusion lung scan). (From James, A. E., White, R. I., Cooper, M., and Wagner, H. N.: Radiology, 100:191, 1971.)

INTERPRETATION: Alveolar pulmonary edema. The focal perfusion defects differ from those present in interstitial pulmonary edema but correspond to the alveolar densities on the chest radiograph. The fluid in the alveoli prevents distribution of radioactivity to those areas.

PROBLEM

Capers Strangefellow, a 51 year old butler, complained of feeling "out of sorts" and experienced diffuse right chest pain. He had a nonproductive cough, temperature of 103.4° F, and a white blood count of 11,300, predominantly neutrophils.

Initial chest radiograph in the emergency room was of poor technical quality and was interpreted as probably normal. The morning after admission he had a perfusion lung scan and repeat chest radiograph. The anterior and posterior views of the lung scan (Figure 23 *A* and *B*) should be analyzed first. Is the distribution of radioactivity in the right lung the same as in the left? Are the abnormalities focal or diffuse, segmental or nonsegmental? Now look at the chest radiograph (Figure 24). You should again consider what clinical diagnosis his history initially suggested to you.

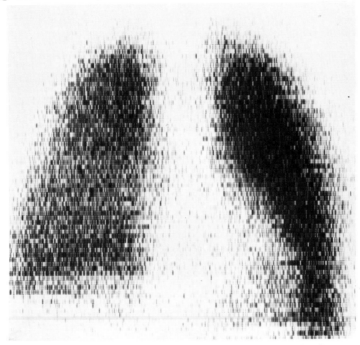

Figure 23 A. *Capers Strangefellow (anterior view).*

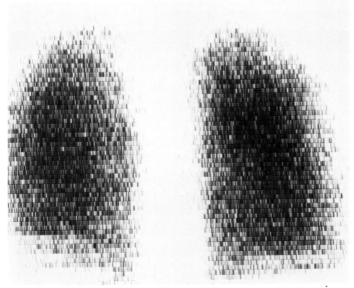

Figure 23 B. *Capers Strangefellow (posterior view).*

Page 27

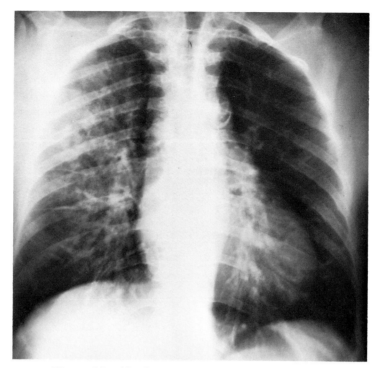

Figure 24. *Mr. Strangefellow's chest radiograph.*

INTERPRETATION: The anterior and posterior views of the perfusion lung scan reveal a generalized decrease in radioactivity in the right mid-lung field. No segmental perfusion defects are seen. On the chest radiograph multiple alveolar densities are present on the right, with prominence of the minor fissure.

Diagnosis: In several days the patient began to produce purulent sputum and the pneumonia on the right became evident.

TEACHING POINT: Inflammatory lesions of the lung parenchyma often cause perfusion abnormalities before they become radiographically apparent. The perfusion abnormalities will persist on the lung scan after the chest radiograph has returned to normal. This phenomenon probably reflects that one study depicts a physiological parameter (lung scan), while the other requires structural or anatomical changes (chest radiograph).

PROBLEM

Evelyn Fewison has had many episodes of "heart dropsy." Physical examination revealed dullness to percussion in the bases bilaterally.

The lateral lung scan (Figure 25) should be viewed concomitantly with the right lateral and decubitus radiographs (Figure 26 *A* and *B*). You are given some clue to the problem simply because a right lateral decubitus radiograph was ordered. Does the unusual shape of the perfusion defect correspond to any density or densities you see on the chest radiograph?

INTERPRETATION: Miss E. Fewison has a linear area of diminished radioactivity corresponding in location and configuration to the major fissure. This has been called the "fissure sign" and may be seen in many diseases, including pleural fluid or thickening of the fissure. On the selected chest radiographs fluid is present in the major fissures and costophrenic angles. The lateral decubitus radiograph demonstrates the mobile nature of the "free" pleural fluid.

Diagnosis: Pleural effusion is the cause of the fissure sign.

EXPLANATION: The exact mechanism of the appearance of the fissure sign is not known. It probably results from diminished peripheral perfusion. Fluid interposed in the fissure could certainly increase resistance to blood flow in the subpleural area adjacent to the fissure, and should diminish the amount of radiopharmaceutical entering this area. Physical separation of the lobes by the fluid may well contribute to the appearance of the "fissure sign" in pleural effusion.

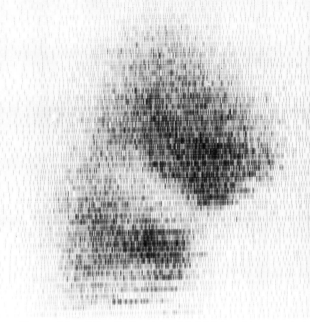

Figure 25. *Miss E. Fewison (right lateral lung scan).*

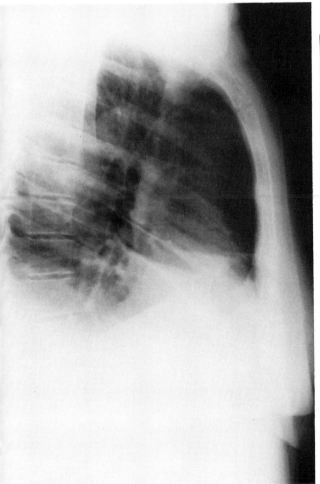

Figure 26 A. *Right lateral erect chest radiograph. (From James, A. E., White, R. I., Cooper, M., and Wagner, H. N.: Radiology, 100:191, 1971.)*

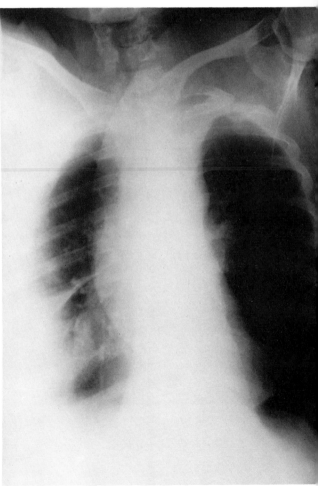

Figure 26 B. *Right lateral decubitus chest radiograph.*

PROBLEM

Alexander Philpott, 41, had alcoholic cardiomyopathy, pulmonary edema and a left pleural effusion. Several abnormal lung scans (not illustrated) were obtained during his hospitalization. Three weeks later a follow-up scan (Figure 27) was obtained to determine if the perfusion defects persisted.

There is an obvious abnormality on the left side which has persisted. How well does the current chest radiograph (Figure 28) agree with the lung scan findings?

INTERPRETATION: The posterior view of the perfusion lung scan shows irregular decreased perfusion to the left lung and a large defect in the left upper lobe.

On the posteroanterior chest radiograph a spherical density in the left upper lobe is present. Is this a lung neoplasm? You remember from the patient's history that he had a pleural effusion. Could post-effusion changes explain the perfusion defects present on the lung scan?

Diagnosis: Loculated fluid in the left major fissure posteriorly, confirmed at fluoroscopy, causing the "pseudotumor" sign.

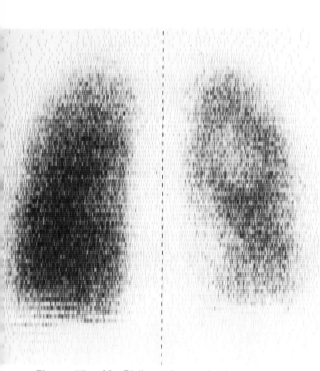

Figure 27. Mr. Philpott (posterior lung scan).

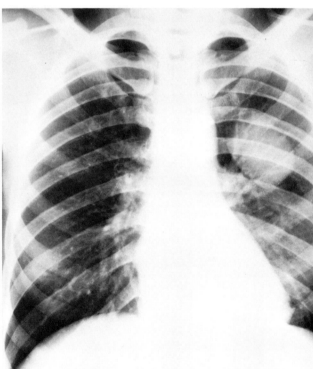

Figure 28. Alexander's chest radiograph.

PROBLEM

Karen Hypere, 46, had rheumatic fever as a child. She has mitral stenosis and insufficiency and has had multiple episodes of pulmonary edema. Recurrent hemoptysis prompted this lung scan.

Only the left lateral (Figure 29) is shown (for some devious motive?). Pay particular attention to the distribution of radioactivity. Compare the amount of radiopharmaceutical in the left upper with that in the left lower lobe. Now examine the chest radiograph and compare the pulmonary vasculature in the upper lobes with the lower (Figure 30). Are the pulmonary vessels as prominent distally as centrally?

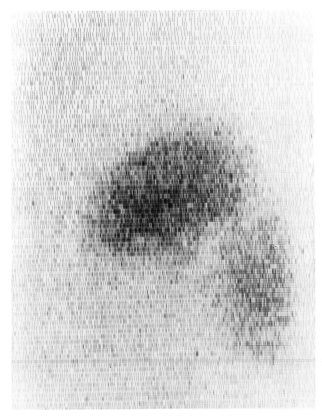

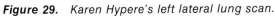

Figure 29. Karen Hypere's left lateral lung scan.

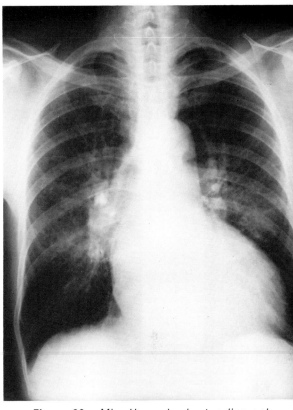

Figure 30. Miss Hypere's chest radiograph.

INTERPRETATION: On the left lateral view cardiomegaly and the "fissure sign" are present. Even more abnormal is the decreased radioactivity to the lower lobe compared to the upper lobe.

An upright posteroanterior chest radiograph shows cardiomegaly with left atrial and left ventricular enlargement. Centrally the pulmonary arteries are prominent and the upper lobe vessels larger than those of the lower lobes. These findings are characteristic of pulmonary venous hypertension with a redistribution of pulmonary blood flow to the upper lobes. A pulmonary angiogram (Figure 31) was performed; this further demonstrates the redistribution (although the patient *is* supine, which accentuates upper lobe flow).

Diagnosis: Pulmonary hypertension, postcapillary type.

TEACHING POINT: In patients with obstruction to left ventricular or left atrial outflow, pulmonary venous hypertension usually results. If this persists, pulmonary arterial hypertension ensues.

Page 31

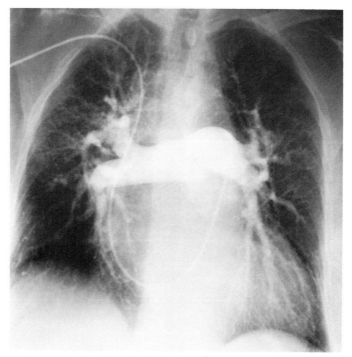

Figure 31. *Pulmonary angiogram on Karen Hypere.*

Pulmonary hypertension is reflected on the chest radiograph by the prominence of the upper lobe vessels and the central pulmonary artery. The redistribution of pulmonary blood flow is manifest on the lung scan by more radioactivity in the upper than lower lobes. The lack of intravascular filling defects and the prominence of upper lobe vessels on the pulmonary angiogram confirms the impression of pulmonary hypertension.

PROBLEM

Candice Bixby, 50, was seen by her family physician for chronic shortness of breath, cough and occasional hemoptysis. She denied vices of any kind. Past medical history was totally positive, but not specific for any known disease disorder. Among her diagnostic studies was this lung scan (Figure 32). She has multiple perfusion defects which are difficult to characterize. Are you really aided by the findings on the chest radiograph (Figure 33)? Well, if you were, you move ahead of us as radiologists.

INTERPRETATION: On the anterior view there is evidence of perfusion defects within the lateral aspect of the right lower lobe, the right apex and the left upper lobe. The inferior border of the radioactivity in the lung appears more irregular than one would expect from respiratory motion alone. These defects are felt to be focal in nature but do not appear definitely segmental in their distribution. There are several etiologies for focal but nonsegmental lesions, but the commonest is chronic obstructive lung disease. The chest radiograph shows several small rounded densities within the left upper lobe and some calcification within the hilar region on the left. This and the slight increase in density at the apices bilaterally are most likely due to chronic granulomatous disease. There is evidence of previous trauma to the right chest posteriorly, since the ribs are irregular. An oblique linear density is present in the right lower lung field arising from the mid-portion of the right hemidiaphragm.

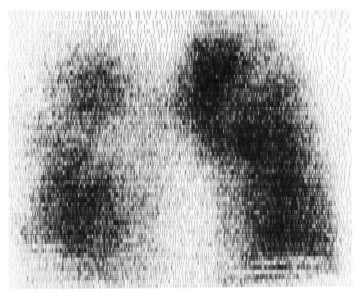

Figure 32. *Candice Bixby (anterior view, perfusion lung scan).*

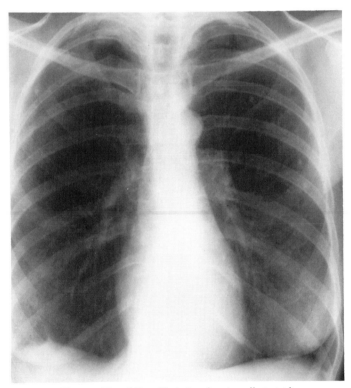

Figure 33. *Miss Bixby's chest radiograph.*

This may represent residual change in the lung from trauma or fibrosis resulting from healing of a previous inflammatory condition.

ADDITIONAL DATA: The patient's pulmonary function evaluation showed values consistent with the diagnosis of obstructive airway disease. However, because of the importance placed upon the history of occasional hemoptysis, a pulmonary angiogram was performed.

The pulmonary angiogram (Figure 34 *A*) shows delay in filling of the vessels bilaterally, more pronounced on the right side. Continued delay of contrast

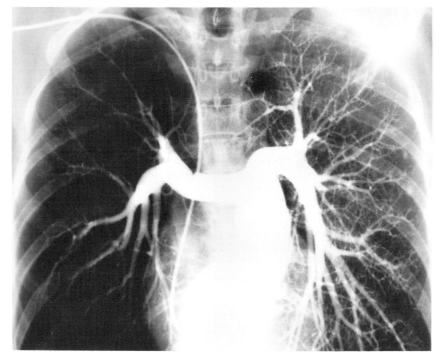

Figure 34 A. *Pulmonary angiogram (early arterial phase).*

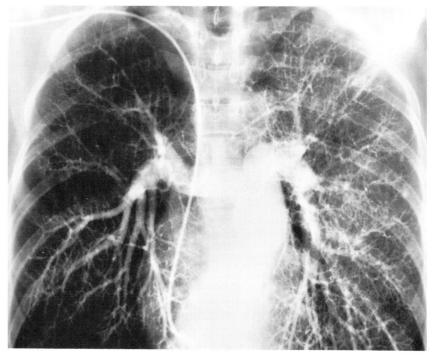

Figure 34 B. *Pulmonary angiogram (late arterial phase).*

flow and tapering of the vessels of the pulmonary artery on that side is present in the later phase (Figure 34 *B*). No intravascular defects are noted within the contrast medium and no definite amputation of vessels is seen; thus, no pulmonary emboli are detected.

This angiogram is consistent with the clinical picture and lung scan diagnosis of chronic obstructive pulmonary disease.

TEACHING POINT: Often there is considerable chronic lung disease that is not readily apparent on the chest radiograph. Fortunately there were changes that suggested this diagnosis here. However, a ventilation lung scan should have been obtained, which may have obviated the pulmonary angiogram. Occasionally patients with minimal chronic lung disease will have small perfusion defects on the lung scan, a normal chest radiograph and normal pulmonary angiogram. Only pulmonary function tests will verify the abnormalities seen on the lung scans.

The ventilatory function of the lung can be assessed by either intravenous injection of a substance that diffuses from the pulmonary vessels to the alveoli, or from inhalation of small particles that pass as far distally as the alveoli. Obstructive lung disease is manifest by abnormalities in the various phases of the ventilatory study. (*Refer to Figure 2* at the beginning of the chapter.) Small airway disease can be seen as trapping of radiopharmaceutical on the "wash-out" portion of the study. Obstruction of large bronchi will result in failure of delivery of the radiopharmaceutical to the affected area throughout the inhalation study.

PROBLEM

Rogers Throckmorton is a 63 year old male with chronic shortness of breath and decreased exercise tolerance. On physical examination there are dimin-

ished breath sounds in the right upper lung. Pulmonary function studies demonstrated a vital capacity of 46 per cent and a forced expiratory volume at one second of 47.5 per cent predicted. The chest radiograph (Figure 35) and lung scan (Figure 36) were obtained. Could you have predicted the perfusion abnormality from the chest radiograph? Pay particular attention to the pulmonary vasculature.

INTERPRETATION: On the chest radiograph there is generalized increase in the pulmonary interstitial markings, which appear irregular. The central pulmonary arteries are prominent bilaterally. In the right upper lung field there is a paucity of vascular markings.

The perfusion abnormalities seen in the lung scan correlate with those that you would have predicted from the chest radiograph. Defects are present in both lungs but almost no perfusion is present in the right upper lobe.

Documenting the regional distribution of chronic obstructive lung disease is often helpful in management of patients with bullous lung disease. There are occasions when surgical removal of nonperfused areas of lung will allow better respiratory function by relieving the compression of relatively uninvolved lung parenchyma.

The inhalation lung scan was obtained to assess regional ventilatory function. On the equilibrium phase there is little radioactivity (^{133}Xe) in the right upper lobe (Figure 37). This information added to that of the perfusion lung scan is most characteristic of large airway obstruction. On the various images of the "wash-out" phase (Figures 38 *A*, *B* and *C*) there is initial retention of the radiopharmaceutical in the left lung at 15 (Figure 38 *A*) and 45 seconds (Figure 38 *B*), but clearing by 80 seconds (Figure 38 *C*).

Diagnosis: Combined large and small airway disease.

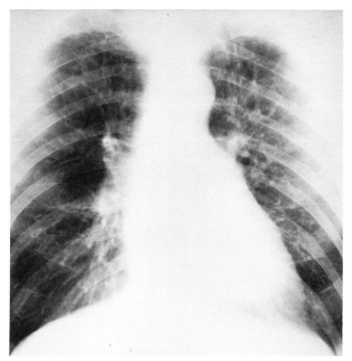

Figure 35. Rogers Throckmorton's chest radiograph.

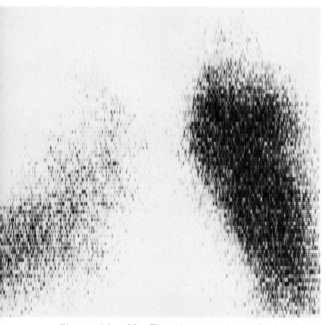

Figure 36. Mr. Throckmorton's perfusion lung scan.

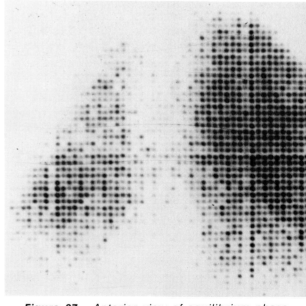

Figure 37. Anterior view of equilibrium phase of inhalation scan taken from computer monitor.

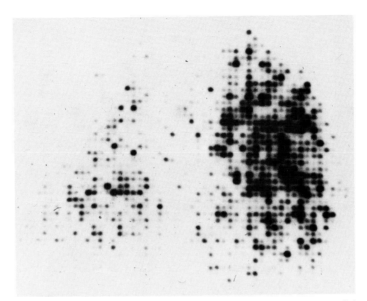

Figure 38 A. *Washout phase of inhalation scan (15 seconds).*

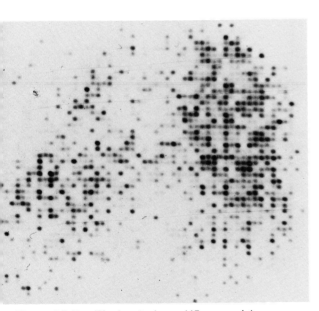

Figure 38 B. *Washout phase (45 seconds).*

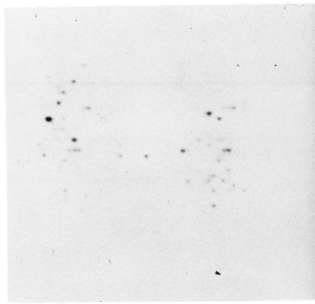

Figure 38 C. *Washout phase (80 seconds).*

PROBLEM

Clarence Gentle, 54, has a longstanding history of chronic bronchitis. He admits to smoking "at least two packs of cigarettes a day" but is able to continue his work as an arc welder. *Mr. Gentle* has had several episodes within the past year of tachycardia, hemoptysis and respiratory distress. This is associated with a continuous nonproductive cough that he relates to smoking. His being seen in the hospital at the present time is the result of an episode of acute chest pain experienced after returning home from work. Compare the abnormalities of the chest radiograph (Figure 39) with those of the perfusion lung scan (Figure 40).

INTERPRETATION: Multiple large perfusion defects are present on the anterior and right lateral perfusion lung scan. There is a smaller perfusion defect in the left upper lung field.

Concomitant chest radiograph shows calcification in the right mid-lung field and hilar regions characteristic of granulomatous disease. The increase in irregularity of the bronchovascular markings, as well as flattening of the diaphragm, is a change seen with chronic obstructive lung disease. However, even more significant is the lack of bronchovascular markings within the entire right upper lung field. This suggests large emphysematous bullae or blebs in these areas. The findings on the lung scan further substantiate the absence of perfusion. Could you predict what the equilibration phase of a ventilation scan would look like?

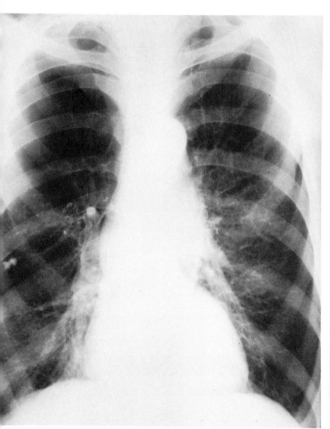

Figure 39 A. *Clarence Gentle's chest radiograph.*

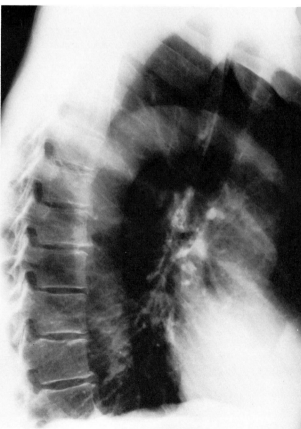

Figure 39 B. *Mr. Gentle's lateral chest radiograph.*

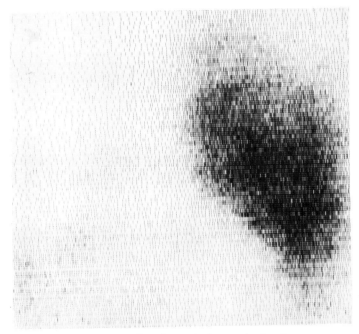

Figure 40 A. *Mr. Gentle: anterior perfusion lung scan.*

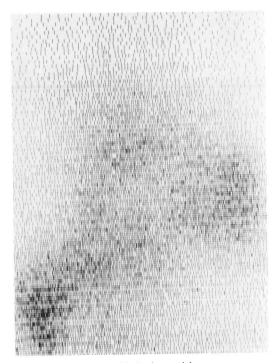

Figure 40 B. *Right lateral lung scan.*

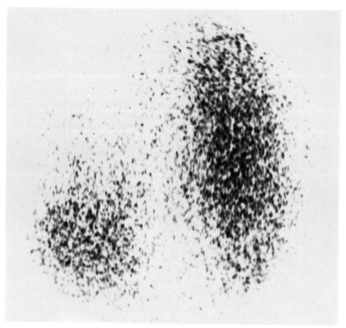

Figure 41. Ventilation scan.

This inhalation lung scan (Figure 41) was obtained with xenon-133. A single view from the equilibration phase is shown. Once again there is lack of radioactivity within the entire right upper lung field, although better ventilation than perfusion is seen at the lung base: *not only is this area not perfused but the airways are obstructed.* This further substantiates the findings on the other diagnostic studies and is characteristic of the lung scan defects one sees with bullous lung disease.

Diagnosis: Chronic obstructive lung disease with bullous changes in the right upper lobe. Were you correct?

PROBLEM

Juana Long, 39, a short-order cook in the Golden Dragon, has complained of many episodes of hemoptysis. Her abnormal chest radiograph (Figure 42) prompted a lung scan (Figure 43). Both the perfusion scan and the chest radiograph are strikingly abnormal. Does the absence of perfusion on the lung scan seem justified by the chest radiographic findings? Can you identify a central pulmonary artery on the left? Are peripheral branches seen?

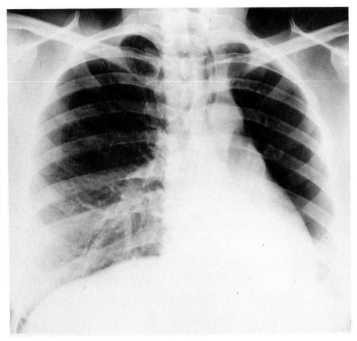

Figure 42. *Juana Long's chest radiograph.*

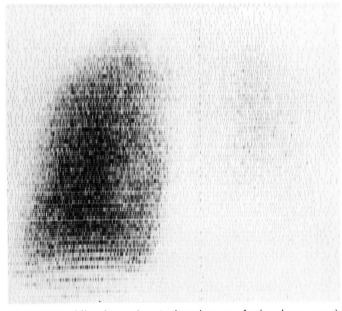

Figure 43. *Miss Long (posterior view, perfusion lung scan).*

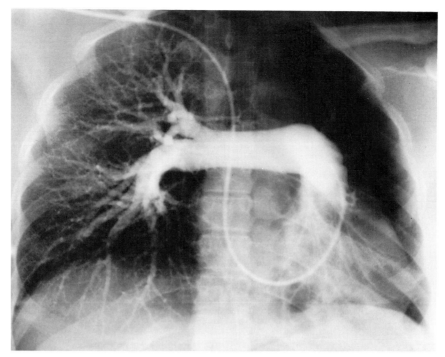

Figure 44. Pulmonary angiogram.

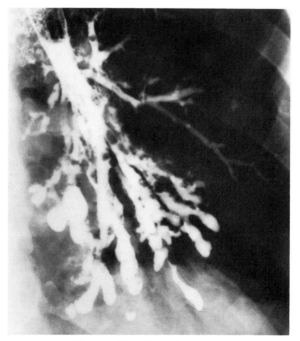

Figure 45. Bronchogram.

INTERPRETATION: Almost total absence of perfusion to the left lung is seen on the scan. The chest radiograph shows almost total absence of pulmonary vessels on the left side. Is there loss of lung volume?

Unilateral absence of perfusion has several causes, which were reviewed on page 16. If you do not remember them, this might be a good time to go back over them.

To establish the etiology a pulmonary angiogram (Figure 44) and bronchogram (Figure 45) were obtained. The pulmonary angiogram reveals almost total absence of vessels to the left lung. Could this be secondary to an abnormality in the lung parenchyma?

The bronchogram (Figure 45) demonstrates saccular bronchiectasis in the left lung and destruction of normal lung architecture.

Diagnosis: Destructive lung disease with secondary vascular changes. One of the well known disorders of similar etiology is Macleod's or Swyer-James syndrome. This syndrome is felt to be due to a previous infection (often adenovirus) leading to parenchymal lung disease and secondary vascular changes. If you did not get this case, try the next one—it's easier, especially if you look carefully at the PA and lateral chest radiographs.

PROBLEM

Longstreet Flint, 66, enters with a history of chronic cough and weight loss. This chest radiograph, (Figure 46) and lung scan (Figure 47) were obtained. Again, almost no perfusion is present on the left side. The chest radiograph explains to some extent the lung scan findings. Is the hilar region on the left prominent? Is there a mass present? If so, what peripheral effect could it have? Could you theorize how these changes could produce unilateral absence of perfusion on the lung scan?

INTERPRETATION: Unilateral absence of perfusion on the posterior view of the perfusion lung scan. But we just said that! The chest radiograph reveals a left hilar mass, left upper lobe atelectasis (you didn't miss it!) and compensatory left lower lobe emphysema. The left hilar mass proved to be a bronchogenic carcinoma. This selective

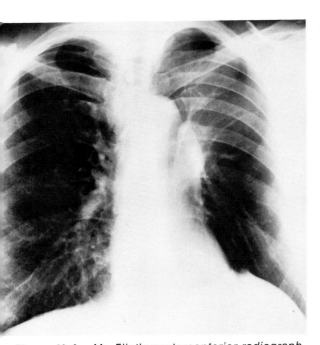

Figure 46 A. *Mr. Flint's posteroanterior radiograph.*

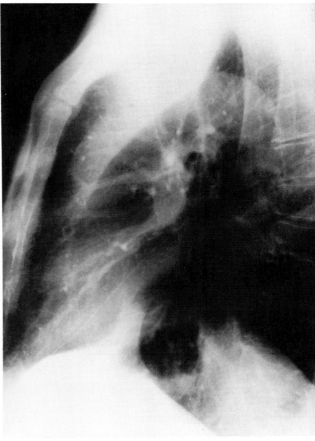

Figure 46 B. *Mr. Flint's lateral chest radiograph.*

(Figure 46 A & B from White, R. I., James, A. E., and Wagner, H. N.: Am. J. Roent., 111:501, 1971.)

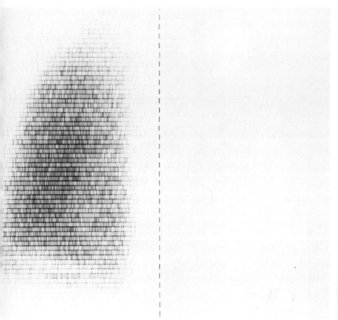

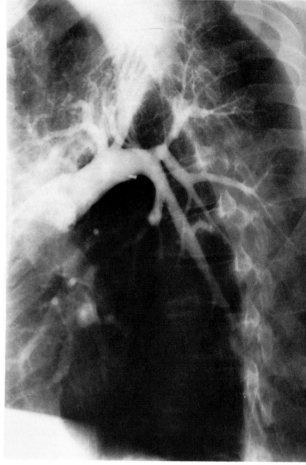

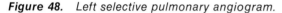

Figure 47. *Longstreet Flint (perfusion lung scan, posterior view).*

(Figures 47 and 48 from White, R. I., James, A. E., and Wagner, H. N.: Am. J. Roent., 111:501, 1971.)

Figure 48. *Left selective pulmonary angiogram.*

pulmonary angiogram (Figure 48) was obtained to see if there was any pulmonary artery invasion to produce the perfusion defect. It shows that the left pulmonary artery is patent and not invaded by the neoplasm. Would you have predicted the angiographic findings?

TEACHING POINT: Central neoplasms often cause profound peripheral perfusion changes without invasion of the vessels. Collapse of the left upper lobe increased resistance to blood flow, as did compensatory emphysema in the left lower lobe. These changes may be reflected on the lung scan as absence of radioactivity in a particular area.

PROBLEM
Gwendolyn Overide, a 14 year old with congenital heart disease, had palliative surgery in 1966 and again in 1967. She

returns for evaluation of the surgical procedure. The combination of the posterior perfusion lung scan (Figure 49 A) and chest radiograph (Figure 49 B) will give some insight into the patient's problem.

There is irregular distribution of the radioactivity in the lungs, with a perfusion defect in the right upper lung. What do you suppose the paired structures are in the abdominal area? You are absolutely right in thinking anatomically because these are, indeed, the kidneys. If the kidneys visualize in a procedure in which the radiopharmaceutical should be trapped in the first capillary bed that they reach, how did they get into the renal arterial circulation from an intravenous injection in the right arm? As I am certain you have reasoned out by now, they passed from right to left through an intracardiac shunt. However, we must explain, from

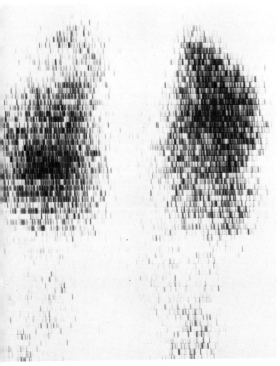

Figure 49 A. *Miss Overide (perfusion lung scan, posterior view).*

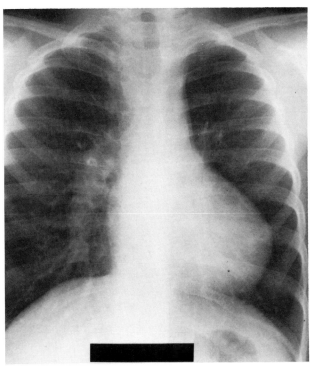

Figure 49 B. *Miss Overide's radiograph.*

the history and the radiographic findings, the perfusion defects noted on the lung scan.

INTERPRETATION: The ribs on the right side appear irregular on the chest radiograph. The fifth rib on the left is minimally irregular. *Gwendolyn's* pulmonary vasculature centrally on the right is increased, but the left does not appear decreased and the aorta is on the left side. The heart is "boot shaped," as the left ventricle is rotated upward by right ventricular enlargement. Following surgery it is difficult from the chest radiograph to know that this was a tetralogy of Fallot.

The patient was known to have had a tetralogy of Fallot, however, and had a Blalock-Taussig anastomosis on the right side in 1966. This was found not to function, and a left subclavian to pulmonary artery anastomosis was performed on the left side in 1967.

EXPLANATION: The perfusion defect within the right upper lung field might

be either from the "wash-out" effect of a functioning shunt, trauma to the right upper lobe during the surgery, an associated peripheral pulmonary artery stenosis that is known to occur with this congenital heart defect, or via bronchial collaterals if the right B–T anastomosis is occluded. If a subclavian to pulmonary artery anastomosis is patent, radiopharmaceutical will often be seen in the opposite lung. This is due to the fact that the arterial blood which is flowing from the shunt does not contain radioactivity from an intravenous injection. Since this is a high pressure system relative to the pulmonary artery, radiopharmaceutical will be physiologically shunted into the lower pressure system opposite the anastomotic shunt. Therefore, this modality gives us a simple, innocuous diagnostic study to evaluate shunt function. For specific anatomical details as to the cause of a nonfunctioning shunt, an angiogram must be performed.

PROBLEM

Galsworthy Glenn, 9, comes to our hospital for (1) evaluation of his shunt procedure and (2) determination of the lung perfusion supplied by his pulmonary arteries. *Master Glenn* had congenital cardiac abnormalities, including pulmonic stenosis. This first lung scan (Figure 50 A) was performed by injection of the radiopharmaceutical intravenously in the right *arm*. Could a common palliative shunt procedure explain the unusual distribution of radioactivity?

The second lung scan was obtained after an intravenous injection of radiopharmaceutical into a *leg* vein (Figure 50 B). For some reason the left lung is now perfused. Could the injection site have made this great a difference? Remember that with the arm injection radiopharmaceutical traveled toward the heart via the SVC, and with the leg injection it passed toward the heart via the IVC.

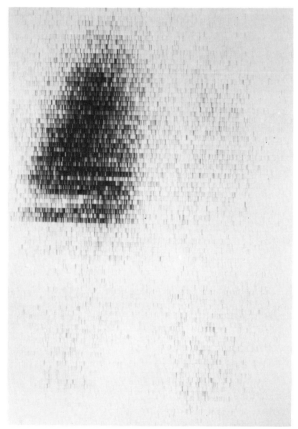

Figure 50 A. *Glenn: Right arm injection. (Figure 50 A, B & C from DeLand, F. H., and Wagner, H. N.:* Atlas of Nuclear Medicine, *Vol. 2, 1970.)*

INTERPRETATION, EXPLANATION PLUS FAITH, AND PROOF: *Galsworthy* had a Glenn operation, which is an end-to-end anastomosis of the superior vena cava (SVC) and the right pulmonary artery. Therefore, with a right arm injection the radiopharmaceutical enters the right lung without passing through the heart. When the radiopharmaceutical is injected into the leg vein it enters the right side of the heart and passes out the pulmonary artery as well

as the aorta. Therefore, the radioactivity is distributed to both lungs (the right may be by bronchial collaterals). Those paired structures are the kidneys (another intracardiac shunt no doubt!)

So that we could end this section on a "moment of truth," we placed a catheter in the superior vena cava and injected contrast into the right pulmonary artery (Figure 50 C): yes it's a Glenn operation for sure—the anastomosis is delineated.

Page 46

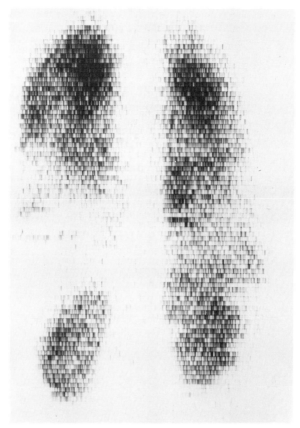

Figure 50 B. *Glenn: Leg injection.*

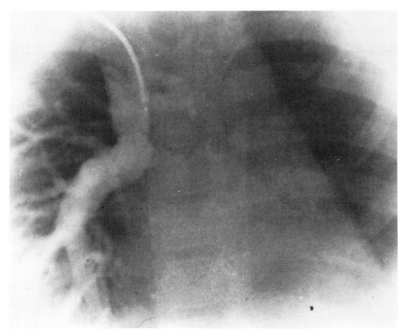

Figure 50 C. *Pulmonary angiogram.*

CHAPTER II

HEART

CARDIAC STUDIES

Radionuclide evaluation of the heart has received increased attention recently as a result of the development of stationary imaging devices such as scintillation cameras in which the entire field of interest can be viewed simultaneously. The development of radiopharmaceuticals with a short half-life allows injection of a bolus which contains radioactivity in multimillicurie amounts. From these developments a new cardiac study, which has been termed *radionuclide angiocardiography,* has been instituted. This simple, safe technique allows investigation of the intracardiac dynamics to diagnose patients with congenital and acquired heart disease and can be used as a screening procedure to select appropriate patients for cardiac catheterization.

Injection of radiopharmaceuticals which are confined to the intravascular compartment will delineate the intracardiac blood pool. This is, of course, useful in the diagnosis of patients with pericardial effusion.

Radiopharmaceuticals which specifically accumulate in myocardial muscle have been sought for some time. The ability to directly image viable myocardial muscle would prove to be of great clinical usefulness in the diagnosis and management of myocardial infarctions and cardiac neoplasms and in determining the success or failure of myocardial revascularization procedures.

INTERPRETATION OF CARDIAC IMAGES

For a radionuclide angiocardiogram a large bolus of radioactivity is "traced" as it passes through the chambers of the heart and the great vessels. From an arm injection the bolus is seen first in the superior vena cava, right atrium, and right ventricle (Figure 51, 1.0 sec.). Then radioactivity passes into the lungs (Figure 51, 3.1 sec.). Following return of pulmonary venous blood the left heart fills and is outlined by radioactivity (Figure 51, 3.5 sec.). Finally,

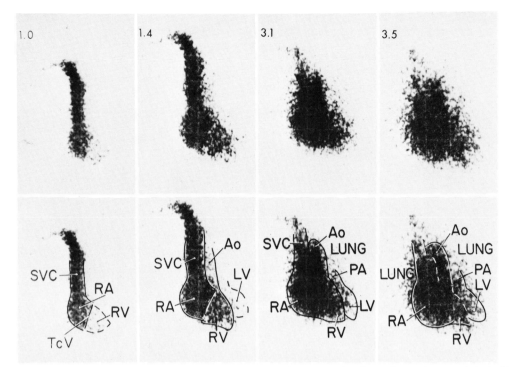

Figure 51. *Anterior view of radionuclide angiocardiogram (duplicate lower images labeled).* *(From Wesselhoeft, H., Hurley, P. J., Wagner, H. N., and Rowe, R. D.:* Circulation, XLV:77–91, *1972.)*

the aorta and great vessels are visualized. These sequential images may be recorded on 35 mm. or 70 mm. film, or 8 mm. movies and give the continuum of observation necessary to detect intracardiac shunts, defects and selective chamber enlargement.

A blood pool study to determine the presence or absence of a pericardial effusion is very reliable, if positive, but somewhat insensitive; that is, we miss small pericardial effusions! The radiopharmaceutical is contained within the cardiac chambers and in the lung and liver (Figure 52 A). Increased separation of the intracardiac radioactivity from that in the lung laterally and in the liver inferiorly is evidence for enlargement of the pericardial space, usually due to pericardial effusion (Figure 52 B, same patient with pericardial effusion). Separation of liver from cardiac blood pool is an unreliable sign when present in the absence of other findings. Comparison of the heart size on a chest radio-

graph (without magnification) and the size of the radionuclide intracardiac blood pool is useful in the diagnosis of pericardial effusion. If the fluid accumulation is great, a "halo" will be present surrounding the heart (Figure 52 B) and appearing to "elevate" the pulmonary arteries. If only a left-sided separation is present, this may represent myocardial hypertrophy (Figure 52 C). Oblique images can be helpful in this differentiation, as they will demonstrate the thickened interventricular septum that accompanies myocardial hypertrophy. (See composite drawing, Figure 53.)

The blood pool study is complementary to the carbon dioxide or contrast injection into the right atrium for the detection of pericardial effusion; the latter are accurate and specific tests but are not without some patient risk and discomfort. The isotope study is not as sensitive but is better tolerated by patients and simpler to perform.

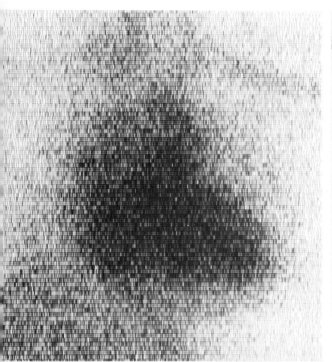

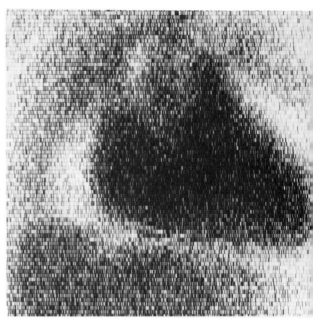

Figure 52 B. *Intracardiac blood-pool study: Pericardial effusion.* (From Hurley, P. J., Wesselhoeft, H., and James, A. E.: Seminars in Nuclear Medicine, 2:365, 1972.)

Figure 52 A. *Intracardiac blood-pool study: Normal.*

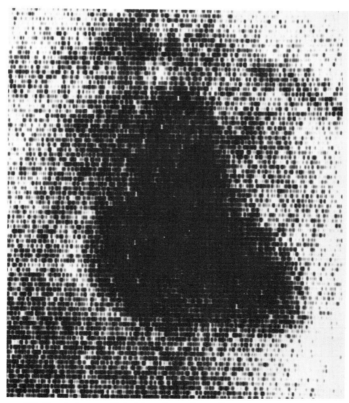

Figure 52 C. *Intracardiac blood pool study: Myocardial hypertrophy.*

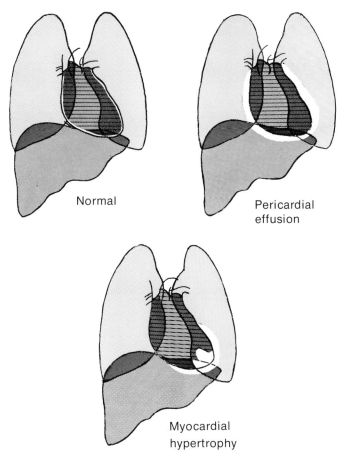

Normal

Pericardial
effusion

Myocardial
hypertrophy

Figure 53. *Intracardiac blood-pool imaging.*

Myocardial Imaging

Direct visualization of myocardial muscle by a radiopharmaceutical that selectively accumulates there would be a monumental achievement. Some progress has been made in this most promising area. The left ventricle is imaged (usually by ^{42}K, ^{43}K or ^{129}Cs intravenously or coronary injection of ^{131}I macroaggregated albumin) as a dense area of homogeneous accumula- tion of radioactivity (Figure 54). Areas of lack of myocardial perfusion are seen as "negative" defects (Figure 55). In this figure a large avascular area is seen which corresponds to the obstruction to contrast flow (arrow) on the coronary angiogram. These may represent in- farcts, or areas of previous myocardial injury that have been repaired by fibrous healing. The clinical history will be of great assistance − isn't it always!

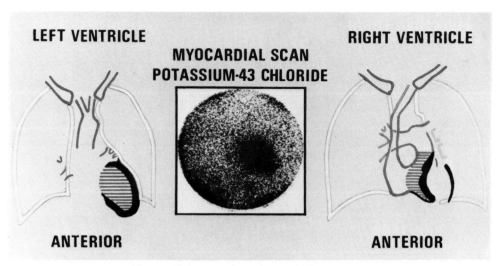

Figure 54. *Myocardial scan: Anterior and slightly obliqued normal. (Courtesy of Dr. Malcolm Cooper.)*

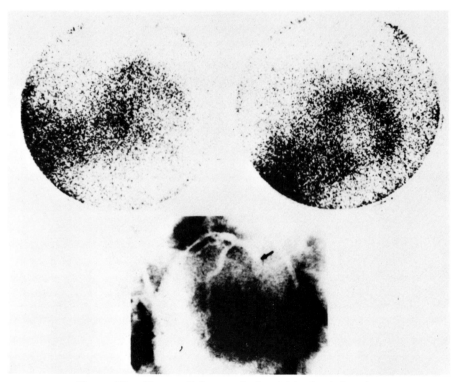

Figure 55. *Myocardial scan: Left ventricular infarction. (From Hurley, P. J., Cooper, M., Reba, R. C., Poggenburg, K. J., and Wagner, H. N.: J. Nucl. Med., 12:518, 1971.)*

PROBLEM

Henry H. Core, 57, was seen in the emergency room because of shortness of breath and ankle edema. On physical examination there were signs of congestive heart failure and cardiomegaly. The electrocardiogram showed evidence of myocardial ischemia. Because of "questionable diminished heart sounds" and low voltage on the ECG, a blood pool cardiac scan was obtained (Figure 56). The differential diagnosis was between a significant pericardial effusion, cardiomegaly and possibly a large ventricular aneurysm.

First, examine the anterior cardiac scan (Figure 56) and anteroposterior chest radiograph (Figure 57, made so that cardiac silhouette is not magnified). *The radiopharmaceutical pool should be 80 per cent as wide as the transverse cardiac dimension on the chest radiograph.* Is it? Now, look for a "halo" or separation from the lung and liver radioactivity. (Compare with Figure 52 *A* and *B*.) Is this a pericardial effusion?

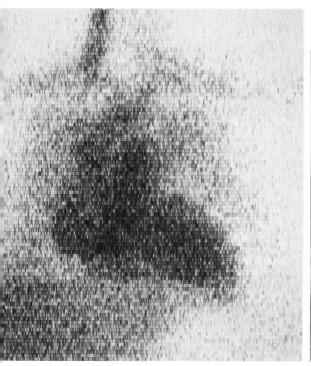

Figure 56. *Anterior blood pool—Mr. Core.*

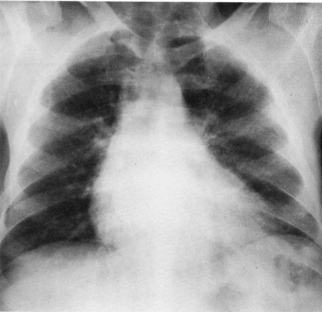

Figure 57. *Anteroposterior chest radiograph.*

ANSWER: The intracardiac blood pool is well outlined on the scan and, in comparison with the concomitant radiograph, is greater than 80 per cent. Thus, the enlargement of the cardiac silhouette appears to be mainly on the basis of left ventricular dilatation. No significant "halo" of diminished radio-activity characteristic of pericardial effusion is seen surrounding the heart. There is no increased space between the radioactivity within the heart and the radioactivity within the liver. For further orientation we have traced in the anatomical structures (Figure 58).

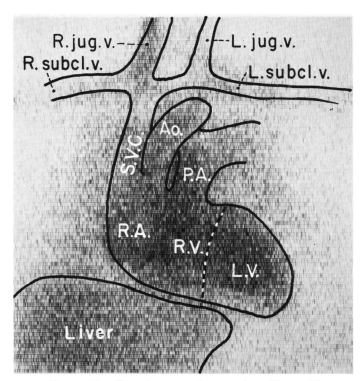

Figure 58. *Drawing superimposed on Figure 56.*

PROBLEM

Regina Queen, 33, is a housewife with chronic uremia. Increasing cardiomegaly has been noted on her physical examination and chest radiographs. A cardiac blood pool study was obtained (Figure 59) to compare the intracardiac radioactivity with the size of the cardiac silhouette on the chest radiograph (Figure 60).

Does *Mrs. Queen* have a pericardial effusion? Could this be myocardial hypertrophy?

INTERPRETATION: It is obvious that there is great disparity between the apparent radiographic size of the heart and the size of the intracardiac blood pool. In addition, the hilar regions appear to be elevated. A surrounding area of decreased radioactivity which appears to encompass the intracardiac radioactivity in a somewhat horseshoe or "halo" fashion is present. There is an increased space between the radioactivity within the liver and that contained within the heart. The fact that the area of diminished radioactivity extends to the right and separates the radioactivity within the lung from that of the intracardiac blood pool mitigates against the diagnosis of myocardial hypertrophy. This is because the right border of the cardiac silhouette is primarily the right atrium, a very thin-walled chamber.

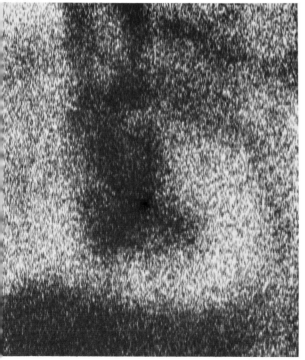

Figure 59. *Mrs. Queen: Intracardiac blood-pool scan.*

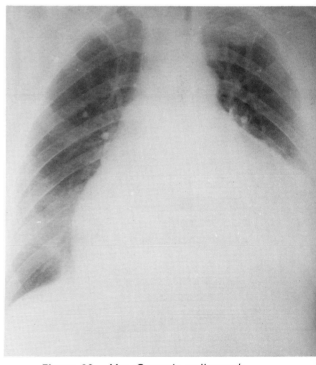

Figure 60. *Mrs. Queen's radiograph.*

Proof: A cardiac angiogram was performed in which radiopaque contrast was intravenously injected (Figure 61). The contrast medium is within the right atrium, right ventricle and pulmonary outflow tract. Comparing the most lateral aspect of the wall of the right atrium with the most lateral aspect of the soft tissue density that makes up the cardiac silhouette, there is a 20-mm. space. *This space should be only several millimeters thick,* confirming the scan impression of a large pericardial effusion.

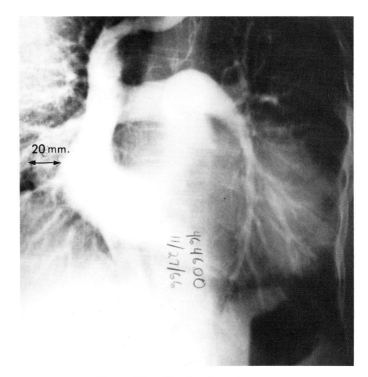

Figure 61. *Contrast angiogram.*

PROBLEM

Gilbert Fuller, a 48 year old alcoholic, entered the hospital following a drinking bout of several days. He is known to have chronic lung disease and cirrhosis. While recovering in the hospital, *Mr. Fuller* had a low grade fever and manifested physical signs of progressive cardiomegaly. Compare the initial posteroanterior chest radiograph (Figure 62) with a subsequent anteroposterior view (Figure 63). His electrocardiogram showed no evidence of a myocardial infarction. There was slightly increased voltage. Because of the findings of increasing heart size with the suspicion of bilateral pleural effusion, an intracardiac blood pool scan was obtained (Figure 64). What would you feel is the basis of his cardiomegaly? Compare with Figure 63.

INTERPRETATION: The intravascular cardiac pool appears to conform to the general shape of the cardiac silhouette but is only approximately 70 per cent the size. The hilar regions do not appear elevated and there is no definite "halo" surrounding the heart. Diminished radioactivity is present on the left side but not on the right. However, medially on the left there *is* a defect in the radioactivity of the intravascular cardiac pool in the ventricle. This is seen with enlargement of the interventricular septum. Enlargement and widening of the interventricular septum is present in patients with left ventricular hypertrophy. This patient proved to have hypertrophy of the left ventricular muscle due to acute alcoholic cardiomyopathy.

TEACHING POINT: If there is only a left-sided "halo" surrounding the intracardiac blood pool and the "septal sign" is present, you may be able to differentiate myocardial hypertrophy from pericardial effusion. The increased voltage on ECG didn't hurt either!

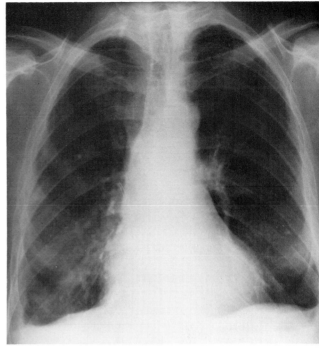

Figure 62. Mr. Fuller's initial chest radiograph.

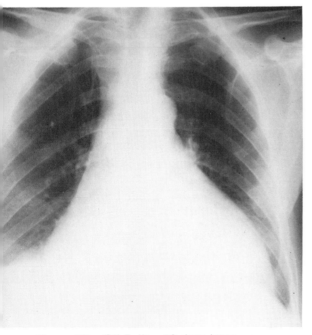

Figure 63. Gil Fuller: 10 days later.

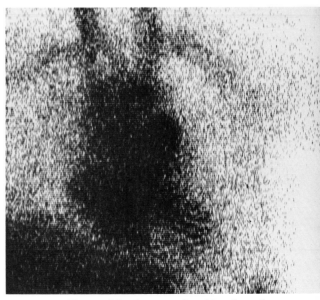

Figure 64. Intracardiac blood pool.

PROBLEM

Aenjina Paectoris, a Greek shipping magnate known for his expensive tastes, suffered "vise-like" anterior chest pain while accompanying his wife on a shopping tour. Several days after his confinement to the intensive care unit, this ^{43}K myocardial scan was obtained in the oblique position (Figure 65). Because this is such a new procedure we include the most abnormal leads of his ECG.

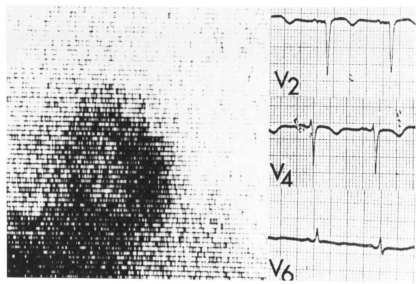

Figure 65. *Myocardial imaging and leads V_2, V_4 and V_6 of ECG. (From Hurley, P. J., Cooper, M., Reba, R. C., Poggenburg, K. J., and Wagner, H. N.:* J. Nucl. Med., *12:518, 1971.)*

Diagnosis: Myocardial infarction, which is present as a large negative defect on the ^{43}K scan and is confirmed by the Q wave and the T wave inversion on the ECG.

TAKE HOME MESSAGE: Myocardial scanning is in its infancy. At present it is not nearly so definitive a diagnostic procedure as coronary angiography, nor so sensitive as the ECG. However, all that is required for this study is a simple intravenous injection of a minute amount of radioactivity. Also, you *directly* image myocardial muscle. The study can be repeated many times; the potential use and great diagnostic implications of this type of study are obvious.

PROBLEM

Bob Reigels, 4 months, is evaluated in our hospital because of cyanosis since birth. Physical examination confirmed this, and also disclosed an accentuated pulmonic second sound that was not split. There was evidence for right ventricular enlargement. Prior to cardiac catheterization this radionuclide angiogram was obtained (Figure 66 A). Trace the passage of radionuclide through the chambers of the heart and notice the origins of the great vessels.

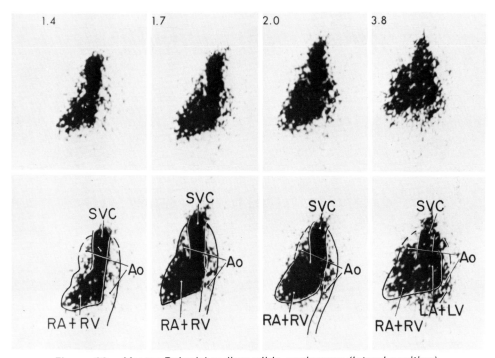

Figure 66. *Master Reigels' radionuclide angiogram (lateral position). (From Wesselhoeft, H., Hurley, P. J., Wagner, H. N., and Rowe, R. D.: Circulation XLV:82, 1972.)*

INTERPRETATION: From the right atrium the radioactivity passes into the right ventricle but not out into the lungs. From the right ventricle radiopharmaceutical goes out into the aorta, and later the left atrium and left ventricle are seen. Almost no activity is present in the lungs. If the right ventricle is connected to the aorta the patient has transposition of the great vessels, as "wrong way" Reigels did.

PROBLEM

Vida T. Redd, 2 years, has exertional dyspnea and occasional syncope. For the past three months the child has had cyanosis. A grade IV systolic murmur with maximum intensity in the pulmonic area is heard. This is associated with a diminished second pulmonic sound and prominent R wave over the right precordium. ECG revealed increased P-wave amplitude in leads II and V_1. A radionuclide angiogram was obtained (Figure 67). Is there any lung activity? Is the persistence of radioactivity in the right heart abnormal?

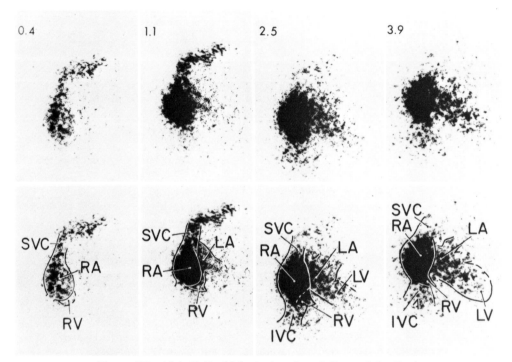

Figure 67. *Vida T. Redd (anterior view, left arm injection). (From Wesselhoeft, H., Hurley, P. J., Wagner, H. N., and Rowe, R. D.:* Circulation, *XLV:82, 1972.)*

INTERPRETATION: Radioactivity passes from the SVC to the large RA (0.4 to 1.1 sec). From the RA the rudimentary RV fills but no activity is seen in the lungs. The LA and LV are then outlined (2.5 to 3.9 sec.) from an intracardiac shunt. This patient had severe pulmonic infundibular stenosis.

TAKE HOME MESSAGE: These examples of radionuclide angiography are difficult to interpret and probably do not absolutely convince you of the clinical utility of this procedure. However, silent movies were not aesthetically pleasing either—so back to the drawing board.

CHAPTER III

LIVER, SPLEEN, PANCREAS

LIVER IMAGING

There are two major types of liver scanning agents, those which go to the parenchymal cells, and colloids (and microaggregates) which go to the reticuloendothelial cells. Thus, the uptake and accumulation of the radiopharmaceuticals employed in liver imaging depend upon either the function of the liver parenchymal cells or the ability of the reticuloendothelial system to engulf colloid particles. Parenchymal cell function is most often assessed by the use of radioiodinated rose bengal. This substance, after intravenous injection, is accumulated within the parenchymal cells and excreted into the biliary system. It then passes, as do iodinated contrast substances, via the common bile duct into the small bowel. Thus, this study produces a functional image of the parenchymal system as well as of the biliary ducts (Figure 68, upper left). Failure of visualization of the radiopharmaceutical in the small bowel can result from either liver disease (Figure 68, lower) or obstruction to the flow of bile for mechanical reasons. If there is obstruction to the flow of bile which is acute and has not altered the parenchymal cell function, rose bengal will be excreted into the common bile duct and you will see it as a dilated structure

containing radioactivity (Figure 68, upper right); no radioactivity will be seen within the small bowel.

Liver disease will be depicted as irregular distribution of radioactivity within the liver image itself without visualization of the bile ducts and absence of radioactivity within the bowel on delayed images (Figure 68, lower).

Since the distribution of the reticuloendothelial cells within the liver is uniform, radioactively labeled colloidal substances, when injected intravenously, will be distributed in a homogeneous manner and delineate the liver (Figure 69, upper). Many different configurations and anatomical variations in liver size and shape have been described. There are normal variations for the divisions of the right and left lobes of the liver, as well as areas of decreased radioactivity in the portal region and gall bladder fossa. The reticuloendothelial system within the spleen and bone marrow will also accumulate the labeled colloid. Normally the spleen is seen as a smaller area of radioactivity that does not contain as much radioactivity as the liver (Figure 69). On views of the liver and spleen in the normal patient, the bone marrow is not well seen.

In liver disease the distribution of

Page 61

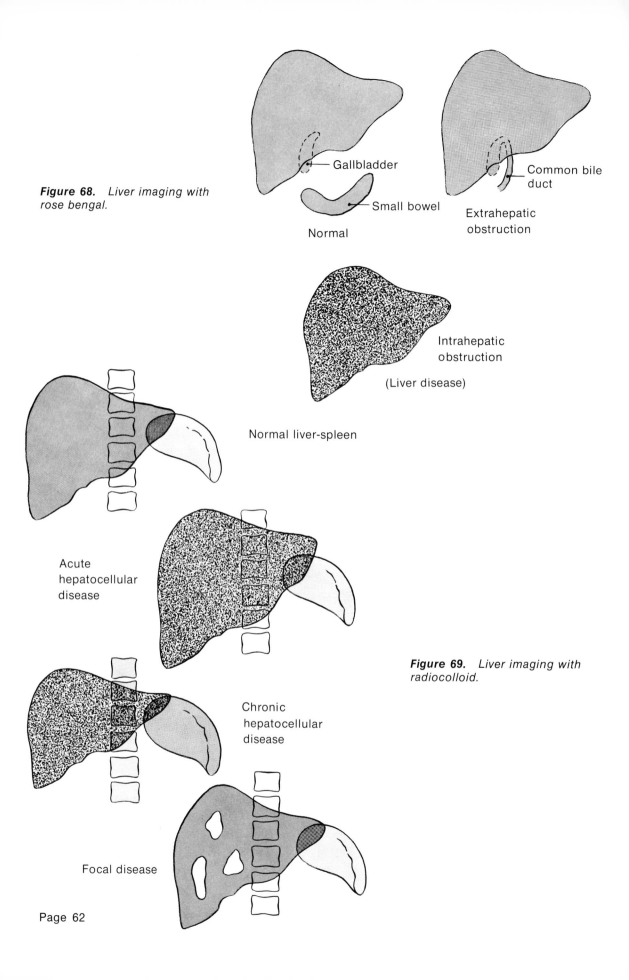

Figure 68. *Liver imaging with rose bengal.*

Gallblader

Small bowel

Normal

Common bile duct

Extrahepatic obstruction

Intrahepatic obstruction

(Liver disease)

Normal liver-spleen

Acute hepatocellular disease

Chronic hepatocellular disease

Figure 69. *Liver imaging with radiocolloid.*

Focal disease

radioactivity within the hepatic structure will be inhomogeneous and irregular (Figure 69, middle two figures); increased radioactivity will occur in both the spleen and bone marrow because the colloidal particles are now taken up there. This is probably because RE cell function in the liver is diminished or portal blood flow is decreased to the liver. Mass lesions within the liver present as negative defects or areas devoid of radioactivity within a field of homogeneous radioactivity (Figure 69, lower).

Multiple views of the liver should be obtained to localize and characterize the size and configuration of the defect. Since the liver is a solid organ, central lesions may not be visualized on a single view but will be detected with greater frequency on multiple views.

Lesions extrinsic to the liver but affecting the liver either by direct pressure or by causing local changes in function within the RES will be manifest as alterations in liver contour. The most common of these are renal and retroperitoneal neoplasms invading or lying adjacent to the liver. Inflammatory conditions such as subphrenic and subhepatic abscesses present as areas of *peripheral* irregularity within the liver radioactivity.

Radiographs should be obtained at the same time as the liver images, with metallic costal markers for orientation. These markers (xyphoid process and costal margin) are extremely helpful in detecting ascites and lesions extrinsic to the liver, and in localizing discrete lesions within the liver substance.

INTERPRETATION OF THE LIVER SCAN

Because the liver is a large solid organ, multiple views in different orientation and degrees of obliquity may be necessary to visualize all the areas optimally (Figure 70 A, B and C, normal anterior, right lateral, posterior recti-

linear scan views, respectively; D, normal camera liver). Because of variations in the surface, a lesion is usually seen on several views before it is considered significant. Along the lower border of the liver, normal negative defects are present in the area of the entry of the portal vein and hepatic artery. Often there is a more lateral defect along the inferior border where the gall bladder rests (Figure 71 A, normal anterior scan, and B, gall bladder study for anatomical orientation). On the lateral margin of the liver image, a linear indentation is occasionally seen which is due to compression from the rib cage. Rarely superimposition of the hepatic flexure of the right colon will cause a defect on the anterior and sometimes the lateral liver scan. Posteriorly the liver is indented by the kidney and adrenal gland. Abnormalities within these structures causing enlargement may increase the defect caused by them on the posterior aspect of the liver.

The upper border of the liver is subject to variation and moulding by the diaphragm (Figure 72 A, anterior; B, posterior, obtained with scintillation camera). Lesions within the right lower lung field and within the pleural space above the diaphragm may cause changes within the upper border of the liver scan.

The left lobe of the liver lies in close proximity to the abdominal aorta and to the upper portion of the lumbar spine. It may be indented by these two structures. There is great variation in the size of the left lobe of the liver and it may be quite small or absent. Occasionally there is a lateral convex indentation of the liver on the left side by either the spleen or the stomach. Medially and on the superior surface of the right lobe of the liver there is sometimes a series of linear oblique defects which probably represent the hepatic veins (Figure 73 A, normal anterior; B, tomographic view). This employs a principle similar to radiographic tomography. Various depths within the solid organ are selected as the plane of optimum resolution.

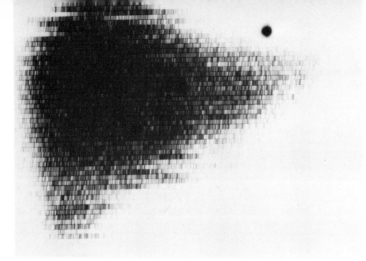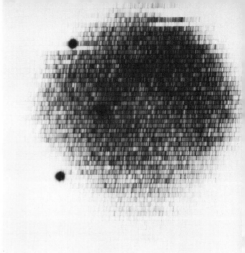

Figure 70 A. *Normal liver: anterior view.*

Figure 70 B. *Normal liver: lateral view.*

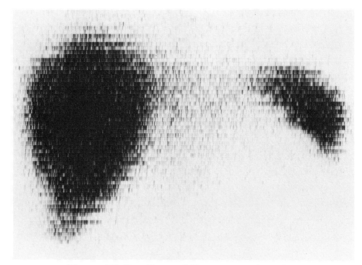

Figure 70 C. *Normal liver: posterior view.*

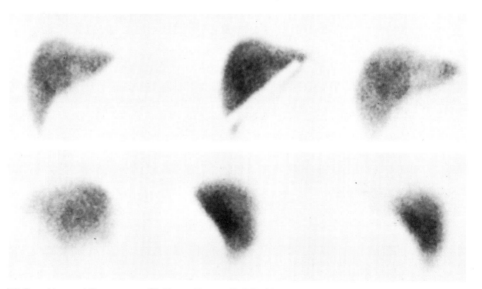

Figure 70 D. *Normal liver scan (⁹⁹ᵐTc sulfur colloid). Upper row, anterior view; anterior view with lead marker on the ribs; and a right anterior oblique view. Lower row, right lateral view; right posterior oblique view; and posterior view.*

Page 64

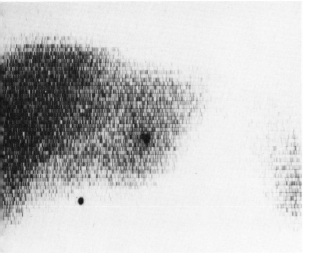

Figure 71 A. *Normal anterior scan.*

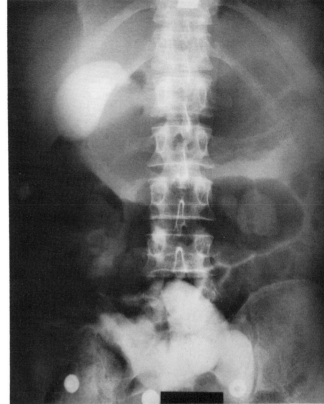

Figure 71 B. *Gallbladder study.*

L   R

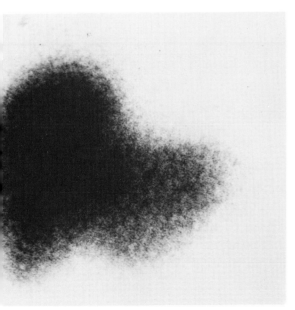

Figure 72 A. *Normal anterior scan (camera image). Demonstrates change in liver shape owing to the diaphragm.*

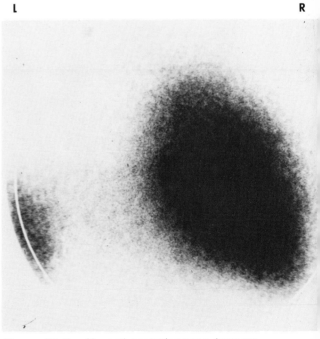

Figure 72 B. *Normal posterior scan (camera image). Again the domed shape of the superior border is present.*

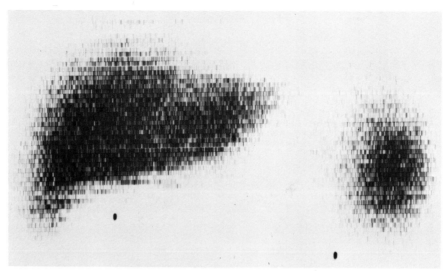

Figure 73 A. *Normal scan, anterior liver.*

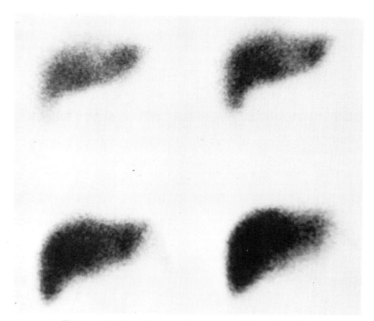

Figure 73 B. *Normal tomographic view; the defect of the superior medial surface is caused by hepatic veins.*

As illustrated previously in Figure 69, parenchymal diseases which acutely affect the liver may cause only enlargement of the organ. However, if the inflammatory component remains for a sufficient period of time, the accumulation of radiopharmaceutical may be generally diminished throughout the liver. Repair of the inflammatory process often consists of regeneration and fibrosis. Areas of regeneration will show normal accumulation of the colloidal particles, but areas of fibrosis will be seen as diminished radioactivity. If the fibrotic process is widespread, large focal defects will be seen which can mimic mass lesions. *Often one cannot distinguish these focal defects from those due to neoplasms, either primary or secondary.*

When the reticuloendothelial function of the liver has been chronically impaired, other areas of reticuloendothelial function such as the bone marrow will accumulate the radiopharmaceutical, and the vertebral bodies and ribs will be visualized. The spleen often becomes enlarged and is seen as a dense area of radioactivity. You will most commonly encounter this pattern in cirrhosis (Figure 69).

One of the most difficult differentiations that must be made on liver scans is to separate the extrinsic lesions that indent the liver surface from those that actually invade the liver itself. These lesions must also be separated from those which arise near the surface of this solid organ. Lesions which merely indent the liver cause a smooth marginal defect in the radioactivity. Those invading the liver cause a very irregular indentation. If you see normal liver parenchyma as an accumulation of radioactivity between the lesion and the surface of the liver on several projections, this usually indicates that the lesion arose within the liver.

Armed with what may be an overwhelming series of possibilities, try some of the problem cases and, if necessary, refer back to the introductory descriptions.

PROBLEM

Jan Czernack, 30, while involved in a heated political debate, was kicked in the right chest. This chest radiograph was obtained (Figure 74). Because of the findings, both a lung and liver scan were included as part of the immediate diagnostic evaluation (Figure 75). After analyzing these studies do you think his problem is above or below the diaphragm?

INTERPRETATION: The chest radiograph shows opacification of the lower right hemithorax. This may be due to effusion, lung hematoma or a ruptured diaphragm with the liver forming the opacity. Whatever the cause of the right lung opacity we must determine if the right lobe of the liver is intact. The lung scan shows lack of perfusion to the right lower lobe, as you would have predicted. However, what we did not expect is that the liver is normal in appearance; par-

ticularly, the superior border is smooth and follows the expected contour of the diaphragm. At laparotomy (not all our colleagues are "believers"), the diaphragm and liver were intact, but there was a right lung hematoma with effusion.

TEACHING POINT: The appearance of the superior border of the liver is an important aid in deciding upon the location of lesions near the diaphragm. Lesions just above the diaphragm will sometimes alter the border of the liver, but the distribution of radioactivity in the liver will usually be homogeneous. Lesions just below the diaphragm cause an irregular distribution of activity in the liver. Often, combination liver-lung scans are very helpful to point clearly to the focus of the patient's clinical problem.

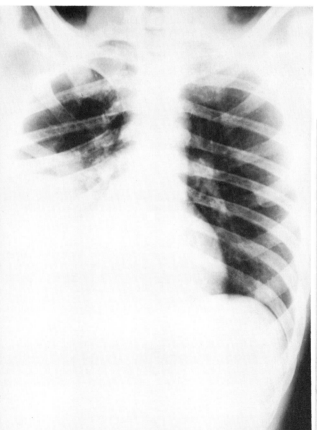

Figure 74. *Jan Czernack.*

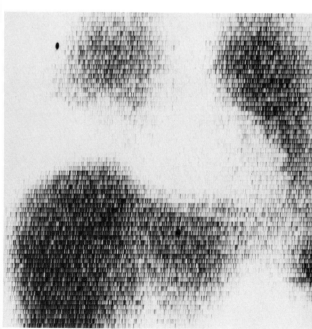

Figure 75. *Liver-lung scan: anterior view.*

PROBLEM

Heinrich von Leichtoffen, 71, sought the assistance of his physician because of sudden right upper quadrant abdominal pain and cough. When he was seen in the hospital, his temperature was 103° F., and he had a white blood cell count of 14,000. Because of the right upper quadrant pain, a liver scan was obtained (Figure 76, anterior, and 77, right lateral). Again your attention is directed to the superior border of the right lobe of the liver.

INTERPRETATION: There is an unusual configuration, as the superior border of the liver is flattened. *Flattening of the liver is seen with chronic lung disease with low horizontal diaphragm, inflammatory disease within the pleural space, pleural effusion and masses in the lower lobe of the right lung.* Subphrenic inflammatory conditions, and conditions involving the superior aspect of the liver *primarily,* do not have this smooth appearance. Inflammatory subdiaphragmatic conditions alter the reticuloendothelial function of the liver superiorly and decrease the uptake of the radioactive colloid. Do the radiographic findings (Figure 78) and the clinical history suggest which of the possible explanations is the most probable?

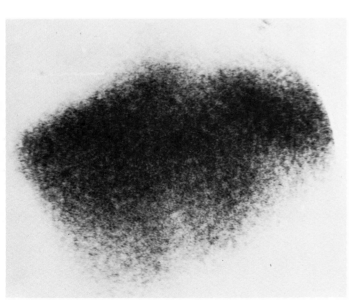

Figure 76. *von Leichtoffen, anterior.*

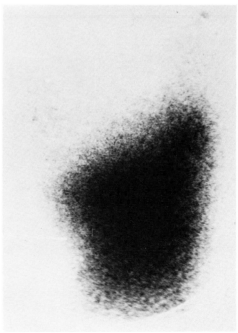

Figure 77. *Right lateral colloid scan.*

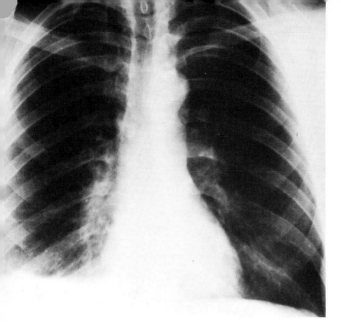

Figure 78. von Leichtoffen's chest radiograph.

ANSWER: The chest radiograph shows a right lower lobe pneumonitis and effusion on that side.

Diagnosis: Pneumonitis, right lower lobe, and effusion.

PROBLEM

Fielding Jones, 23, was involved in a riot, during which he was wounded. There was generalized gunfire; he was a nonselected recipient. When *Mr. Jones* entered the emergency room, his initial hematocrit was 36, but within several hours it was found to be 29. In the interim, a liver scan was obtained with radiocolloid (Figure 79). How does the upper border of the right lobe in *Mr. Jones* differ from those in the two preceding patients? Does the chest radiograph offer any clues (Figure 80)?

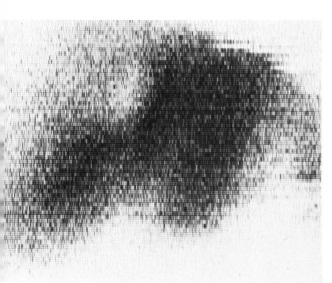

Figure 79. Mr. Jones' anterior liver scan.

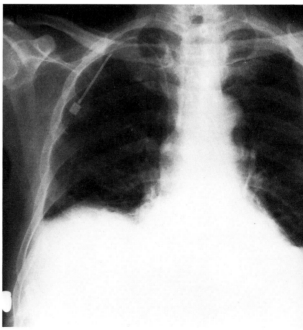

Figure 80. Fielding Jones' radiograph.

ANSWER: On the liver scan there is irregularity and a focal defect of the superior portion of the right lobe. The remainder of the liver appears normal except that the left lobe is larger than usual.

The concomitant chest radiograph (Figure 80) shows soft tissue emphysema bilaterally, as well as bilateral pleural effusion. *Mr. Jones'* right hemidiaphragm appears elevated.

On the abdominal radiograph (Figure 81) a metallic density is present, representing a large bullet fragment in the right upper quadrant. Because of this and the changes within the right lower lung field, it was felt that this patient had lung parenchymal *and* hepatic trauma.

At operation *Mr. Jones* had contusion of the right lower lung, laceration of the right hemidiaphragm, and contusion and a large hematoma in the upper portion of the right lobe of the liver.

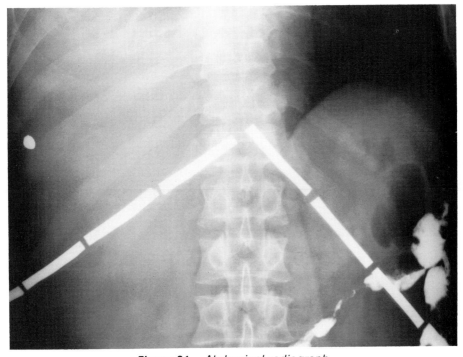

Figure 81. Abdominal radiograph.

PROBLEM

Laura Nevus, a 26 year old secretary, had a pigmented lesion excised from her right lower leg seven months prior to admission. Her first chest radiograph (Figure 82) was obtained at that time.

Miss Nevus is now complaining of generalized malaise, lethargy and pain in her right upper quadrant. Her BSP retention is 24 per cent. On physical examination, diminished breath sounds were present in her right lower lung. A liver scan (Figure 83, anterior (A) and right lateral (B) and repeat chest radiographs (Figure 84 A and B) were obtained. How are the changes on the two chest radiographs explained by the liver scan?

INTERPRETATION: On the anterior and right lateral views of the liver scan, a large area devoid of radioactivity within the right lobe and affecting the left lobe is present. This appears to be a single large lesion with no normal liver in that area. The remainder of the liver is normal and no splenomegaly is present.

CLUE: Although hepatomas and primary tumors of the liver may arise in a normal liver, you will often see the characteristic changes of cirrhosis accompanying hepatoma. Large solitary secondary metastases in the liver may derive from several types of primary neoplasms.

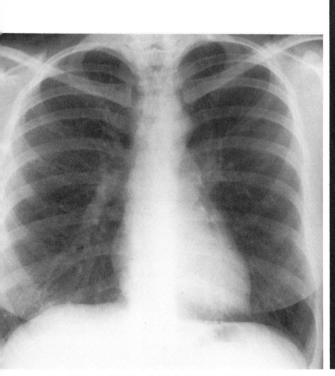

Figure 82 A. *Initial chest radiograph, postero-anterior.*

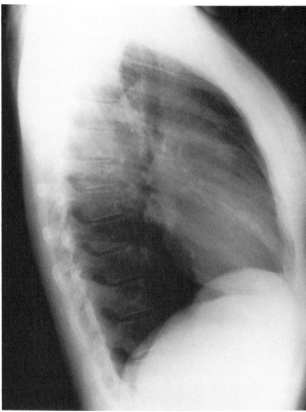

Figure 82 B. *Lateral chest radiograph.*

The radiographs at the time of the patient's surgery and on the present admission prove helpful in the differential diagnosis. The chest radiograph at the time of previous surgery is normal, but the present radiograph shows an elevation of the right hemidiaphragm with displacement of the heart to the left.

In the left upper lobe of the lung there are several densities that were not present on the previous radiograph. A density is also seen overlying the anterior fourth rib on the right side. These abnormalities are most probably metastases.

Diagnosis: Metastatic melanoma from the previously excised primary on the right leg.

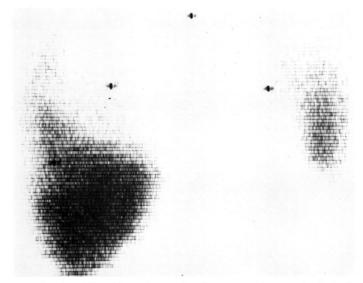

Figure 83 A. *Miss Nevus' anterior liver scan (second admission).*

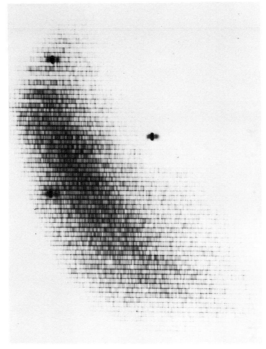

Figure 83 B. *Miss Nevus' right lateral scan.*

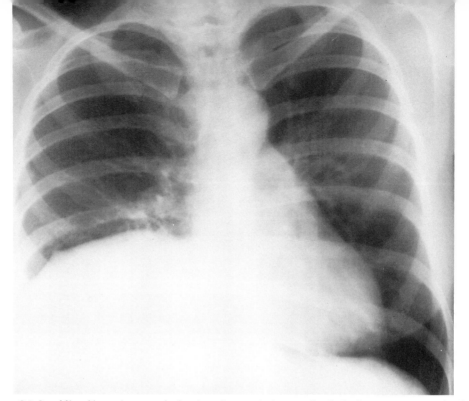

Figure 84 A. *Miss Nevus' second chest radiograph (second admission seven months later).*

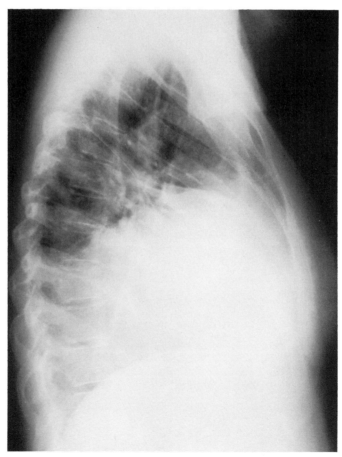

Figure 84 B. *Miss Nevus' lateral radiograph.*

PROBLEM

Belinda Maas, a 47 year old housewife, is being evaluated for an acute depression. Her BSP retention was 15 per cent. On physical examination the spleen was palpable and questionably enlarged. A mass was palpated in the upper abdomen in the mid-line. Because of these findings, a liver scan was obtained (Figure 85 A and B).

These anterior and posterior views are shown for your analysis. Do you think the splenic radioactivity is normal? The posterior view shows a distinct abnormality not depicted by the anterior. Can you localize it? Does it arise within the liver?

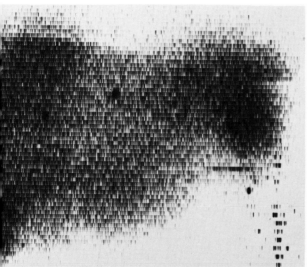

Figure 85 A. *Mrs. Maas' anterior colloid liver scan.*

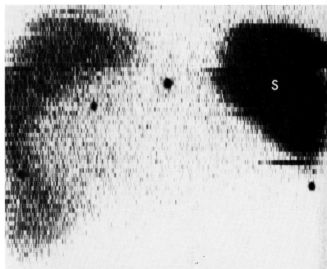

Figure 85 B. *Mrs. Maas' posterior view.*

INTERPRETATION: The anterior colloid scan shows diffuse enlargement of the liver with slight splenic enlargement. The left lobe of the liver appears to be selectively enlarged. On the posterior scan, however, there is a striking abnormality involving most of the right lobe. There was a great deal of discussion as to whether or not this represented an intrinsic mass within the liver, such as a hepatoma. The spleen is definitely enlarged on the posterior view. The "lesion" on the right is noted only on the posterior view and was not seen on the right or left lateral views. Might this posterior indentation of the liver represent a normal structure and, if so, what structure has this shape and lies in this position?

ANSWER: Abdominal radiograph (Figure 86) shows the normal right kidney to lie just in the area of the abnormality on the posterior scan. The configuration and position conform exactly to the defect. This has been seen on a number of occasions and must always be considered when a lesion is present only on the posterior view.

Diagnosis: At exploratory laparotomy there was renal impression on an enlarged liver. The spleen *was* enlarged because of nodal impression on the splenic vein from a previous inflammatory condition, probably granulomatous. (The surgery apparently cured her depression.)

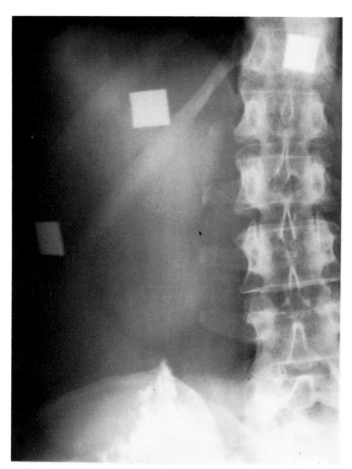

Figure 86. Abdominal radiograph (square densities are lead rib-cage markers).

PROBLEM

Billy Wassacell, 63, entered the hospital with complaint of weight loss and right upper quadrant pain. His liver chemistries were abnormal. A mass was felt in the right upper quadrant on physical examination. Urinalysis revealed microscopic hematuria. A liver scan was obtained (Figure 87 A and B).

There are immediate similarities to the problem of Mrs. Maas, but, thinking anatomically, several important differences are present in addition. Is the defect also seen in the anterior view? Can you detect it on the lateral view? Is the distribution of radioactivity in the remainder of the liver homogeneous? Has it focal defects? Or is it slightly irregular? *None of the above!*

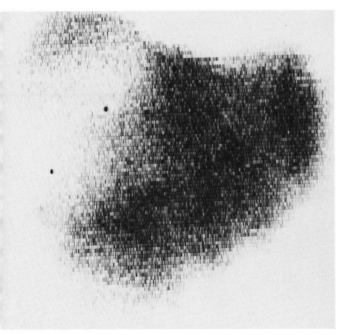

Figure 87 A. *Mr. Wassacell's anterior liver scan.*

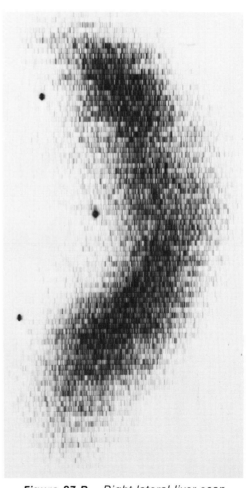

Figure 87 B. *Right lateral liver scan.*

(Figure 87 A, B, D & E from DeLand, F. H., and Wagner, H. N.: Atlas of Nuclear Medicine, *Vol. 3, 1972.)*

INTERPRETATION: On the anterior and right lateral views of the liver scan there is a large mass laterally and posteriorly that involves the right lobe of the liver. No normal liver tissue surrounds the mass. It was believed that the most likely diagnosis was a primary liver neoplasm, but some observers questioned the possibility of an extrinsic lesion pressing upon or invading the liver. Because of the irregular outline of the borders of the radioactivity within the area of the lesion, we reasoned that if this were a lesion involving another structure or organ, it was certainly invading the liver. The most likely diagnosis then would be a renal neoplasm, an adrenal tumor or a retroperitoneal mass invading the liver. How could you evaluate these possibilities radiographically with a single study?

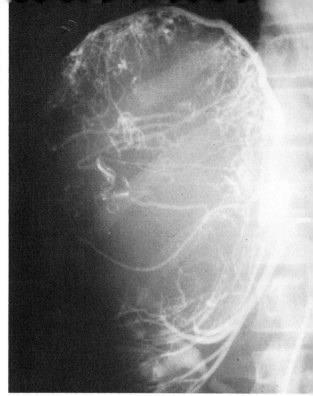

Figure 87 D. *Selective renal angiogram (arterial phas*

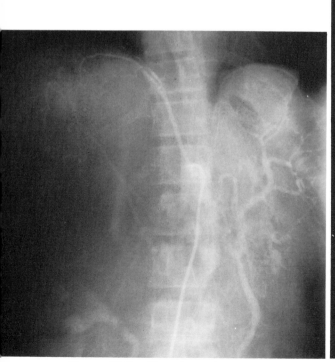

Figure 87 C. *Hepatic angiogram.*

Page 78

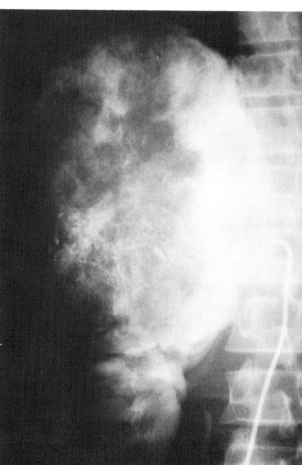

Figure 87 E. *Selective renal angiogram (capillary pha*

ANSWER: Selective hepatic and renal angiography (Figure 87 *C*, *D* and *E*) revealed markedly abnormal vessels within the area of the mass. By selective catheterization of the various vessels supplying this lesion as well as analysis of the capillary phase, this was shown to be a primary renal neoplasm.

Diagnosis: Hypernephroma of the upper pole of the right kidney invading the liver. Therefore, this is an abnormality on the liver scan secondary to a primary neoplasm in an adjacent structure invading the liver.

PROBLEM

Paulette Crampton, age 6 weeks, enters because of respiratory distress. Figure 88 is her admission chest radiograph. An anterior colloid liver scan (Figure 89 *A*) and an abdominal radiograph (Figure 89 *B*) were obtained to determine the position of the liver.

Compare the chest and abdominal radiographs with the liver scan. Where do you think the liver is with regard to the spleen?

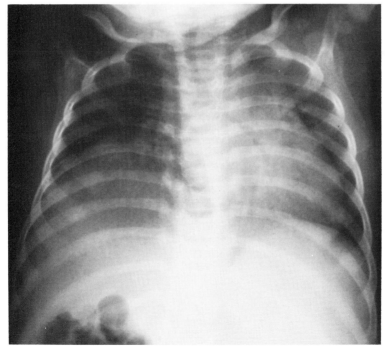

Figure 88. *Miss Crampton's chest radiograph.*

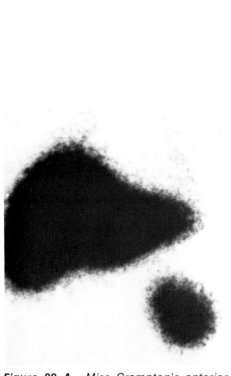

Figure 89 A. Miss Crampton's anterior liver scan (camera view).

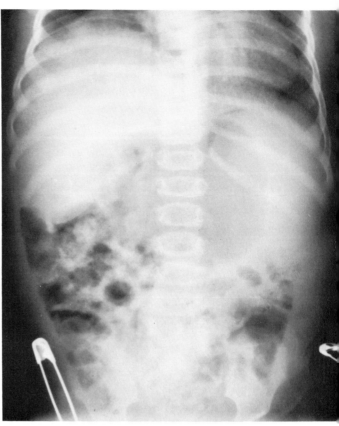

Figure 89 B. Miss Crampton's abdominal radiograph.

INTERPRETATION: The liver in the scan image lies superiorly and is oblique in its orientation. The spleen is rotated inferiorly and somewhat medially because of the displacement of the liver upward.

The concomitant abdominal radiograph shows the liver to lie within the right lower chest and suggests the correct diagnosis. The left upper quadrant density appeared to be the spleen but must be a composite of the gastric fundus, left colon and spleen. The radiograph demonstrates displacement of the cardiac silhouette to the left and ap-

parent elevation of the right hemidiaphragm. If the appearance of the lower lung field had been due to collapse of the right lower lobe with elevation of the hemidiaphragm, would this shift of the cardiac silhouette be present?

Diagnosis: Eventration of the right hemidiaphragm with respiratory compromise on the basis of loss of lung volume due to the presence of the liver within the right chest. Surgical repair was accomplished.

PROBLEM

Miss Flora Roses admitted to an age of 59, but had the appearance of age 95. She was in our hospital because of disorientation, hallucinations and swelling of the abdomen and lower legs. *Miss Roses* was anemic, with a hematocrit of 29 per cent, and had a markedly abnormal liver profile. This liver scan was obtained (Figure 90, posterior view). A number of structures are delineated that are not normally seen. Can you identify them? Is the liver large, normal or small? Compare hepatic and splenic radioactivity.

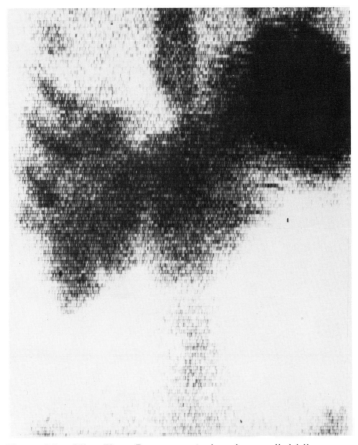

Figure 90. *Miss Flora Roses, posterior view, colloid liver scan.*

INTERPRETATION: On the posterior view of the liver scan, the liver itself is small and there is diffuse irregularity of distribution of the radiocolloid. The series of linear areas of radioactivity that you noted laterally on the right side represent the reticuloendothelial cells within the ribs, and the midline linear radioactivity is in the thoracic and lumbar spine. The very dense radioactivity within the left upper quadrant is the enlarged spleen.

This liver scan has the characteristic findings of cirrhosis. There is enhancement of the reticuloendothelial activity within the osseous structures as well as enlargement of the spleen, probably due to portal hypertension. Biopsy and splenoportogram confirmed these findings.

Diagnosis: Cirrhosis with portal hypertension.

PROBLEM

Archibald Brewer, IV, 43, entered the hospital with an acute gastrointestinal hemorrhage following a rather lengthy cocktail party. Upper gastrointestinal series revealed varices in the distal esophagus and in the gastric fundus. There was a history of previous weight loss, but recent weight gain over the past two to three weeks. This liver scan was obtained (Figure 91 A and B).

There are certain aspects of the history that are compatible with the same diagnosis as that of the last patient. However, the images are different. Could this be another variant of the spectrum of changes seen with cirrhosis? You could probably profit from a review of the introductory remarks on the varied findings seen in cirrhosis.

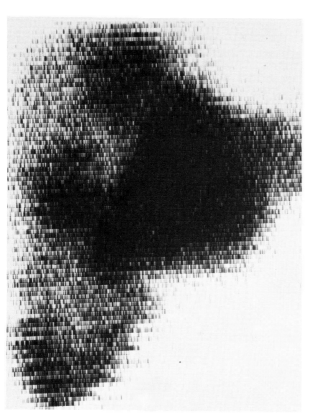

Figure 91 A. *Mr. Brewer, anterior view, liver scan.*

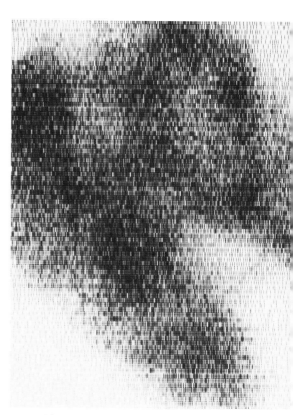

Figure 91 B. *Right lateral liver scan.*

INTERPRETATION: There is diffuse non-homogeneity of the distribution of radioactivity within this solid organ. However, you can see focal lesions laterally on the anterior and right lateral views. Although it was felt that the patient did, indeed, have cirrhosis, the focal nature of the diminished radioactivity increased the probability that the patient might have an associated hepatoma. Therefore, selective hepatic angiography was performed (not illustrated) which showed characteristic signs of cirrhosis. No tumor vessels were seen, however. Because of some remaining uncertainty, the patient had an open liver biopsy which showed marked changes of cirrhosis with large areas of healing fibrosis, but no hepatoma.

TEACHING POINT: Cirrhosis (healing with fibrosis) may cause "pseudotumor" changes, manifest as large focal areas of diminished radioactivity on the liver scan. These may sometimes be indistinguishable from neoplastic masses.

PROBLEM

Brooker Falcon, 51, is a known cirrhotic who enters the hospital because a midline epigastric mass was palpated. He has had a previous splenoportogram which demonstrated portal hypertension; varices were present on barium contrast studies of the upper gastrointestinal tract. A large mass is palpable within the upper mid-abdomen which had not previously been observed. A liver scan was obtained (Figure 92 *A* and *B*). Do you see absence of radioactivity or an enlarged left lobe of the liver to account for the physical findings of a mass? If not, should you probably discount the physical findings as erroneous or re-examine the patient yourself?

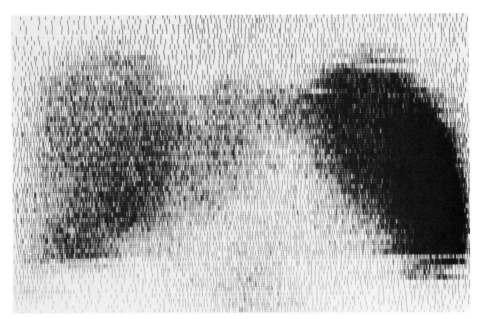

Figure 92 A. *Mr. Falcon, anterior view.*

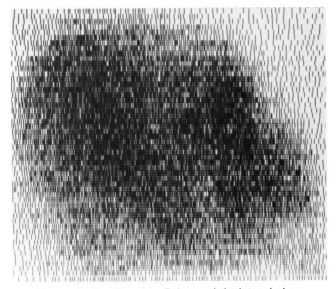

Figure 92 B. *Brooker Falcon, right lateral view.*

INTERPRETATION: The anterior and right lateral views of the liver scan show diffusely irregular radioactivity with homogeneous dense radioactivity in the enlarged spleen. Minimal activity in the spinal region is noted. However, there is little evidence of a mass lesion within the mid-abdomen. The size of the left lobe of the liver appears to be in proportion to the size of the right lobe. This was interpreted, then, as showing classic changes of cirrhosis with splenomegaly.

Because of the continued interest of the clinical staff in the palpable mass within the abdomen, a celiac and selective hepatic angiogram was obtained (Figure 93 A and B).

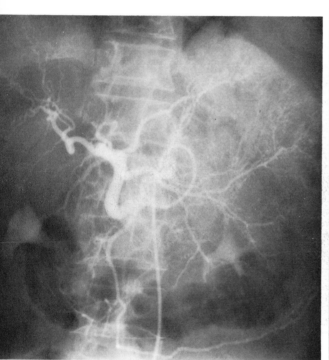

Figure 93 A. *Mr. Falcon, celiac angiogram.*

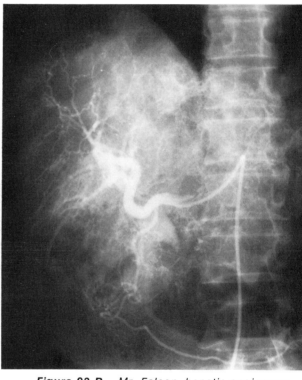

Figure 93 B. *Mr. Falcon, hepatic angiogram.*

ANSWER: There are, indeed, the changes of cirrhosis throughout the liver, with irregularity and a "cork-screw" appearance of the hepatic vessels. However, markedly abnormal vessels in the entire upper mid-abdomen are present both on the celiac and selective hepatic angiograms. At autopsy this was found to be a large hepatoma replacing the entire left lobe and extending into a portion of the medial aspect of the right lobe. The lesion was so large that it had entirely replaced all the normal liver within this area, and no reticulo-endothelial function was present at all. Therefore, the mass itself was not visualized on the liver scan! (In our experience this is a very unusual circumstance.)

PROBLEM

Edith Egress, 46, is being evaluated because of a right upper quadrant mass that was palpated on routine physical examination. Except for the mass, *Edith* has been in good general health. She admits to a 20-pound weight loss in the last three months but has attributed this to voluntary dieting. A liver scan was obtained (Figure 94 *A* and *B*). Does this lesion appear intrinsic or extrinsic?

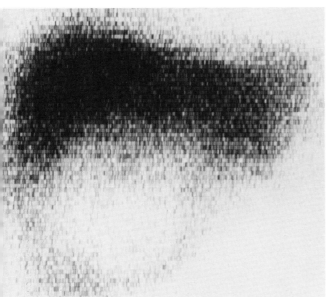

Figure 94 A. *Miss Egress, anterior colloid liver scan. (From DeLand, F. H., and Wagner, H. N.:* Atlas of Nuclear Medicine, *Vol. 3, 1972.)*

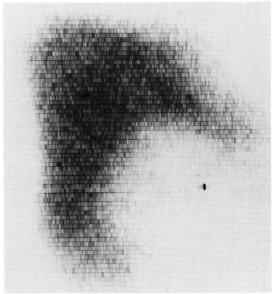

Figure 94 B. *Miss Egress, right lateral scan.*

INTERPRETATION: The anterior and right lateral liver scan reveal a large single area of diminished radioactivity. On the anterior scan some colloid radioactivity is noted surrounding the entire mass. This was believed to represent a large liver neoplasm on the anterior surface of the liver. The celiac angiogram (Figure 95) shows the abnormal vasculature in the liver, with stretching of vessels and abnormal vessels surrounding the neoplasm. Both kidneys appeared normal.

Diagnosis: Hepatoma.

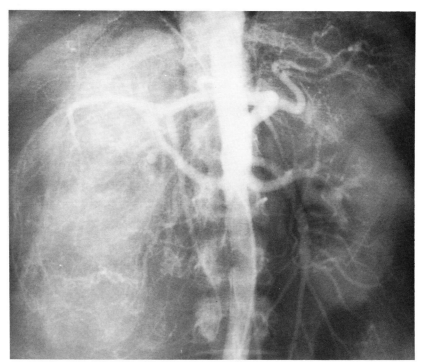

Figure 95. *Celiac angiogram. (From DeLand, F. H., and Wagner, H. N.:* Atlas of Nuclear Medicine, *Vol. 3, 1972.)*

TEACHING POINT: The rim of radioactivity surrounding the lesion on the anterior scan suggests that it was primarily an intrinsic process. Our confidence in this finding would have been much greater had it also been surrounded by radioactivity on the lateral view as well.

PROBLEM

Harold Courvoisier is a three month old child who has jaundice and increased abdominal size. An ^{131}I rose bengal scan was obtained (Figure 96 *A*, 2 hours anterior; *B*, 17 hours anterior).

Remember that rose bengal passes through the liver and biliary system in much the same manner as iodinated contrast agents (Telepaque, Cholografin). Thus, we normally expect to see ^{131}I in the liver parenchymal cells and then in the small bowel via the common bile duct.

INTERPRETATION: On the anterior view at two hours the liver is seen (Figure 96 *A*). There appears to be a mass within the liver in the right lobe involving the inferior aspect. In the hope of detecting the presence of obstruction, a delayed scan was obtained (Figure 96 *B*). At 17 hours the liver radioactivity remains. However, there is a very dense area of radioactivity which now occupies the area of the defect seen on the first scan.

TEACHING POINT: If this were radiographic contrast you might imagine a structure filling on the delayed view. Thinking physiologically with regard to the distribution of rose bengal, this radioactivity might be within the biliary tree, the gall bladder or the bowel. However, since it filled in the exact area of the previous defect on the early liver scan, the gall bladder or a cyst in the area of the gall bladder is most likely.

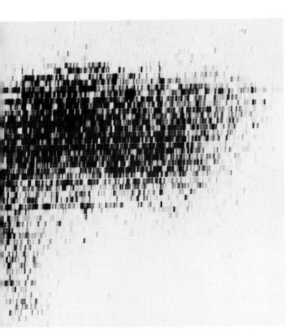

Figure 96 A. *Anterior view, rose bengal scan (two hours).*

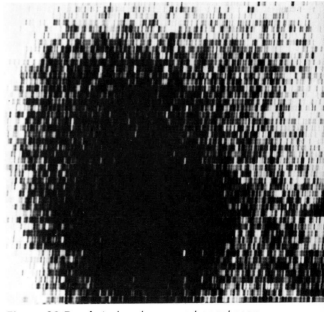

Figure 96 B. *Anterior view, rose bengal scan (17 hours).*

(Figure 96 A & B from DeLand, F. H., and Wagner, H. N.: Atlas of Nuclear Medicine, *Vol. 3, 1972.)*

OPERATIVE FINDING: Congenital chol-edochal cyst.

Sometimes rose bengal studies are not so strikingly abnormal, but if we continue with our physiological bias of interpretation and examine the studies in proper temporal sequence, we can draw many useful conclusions. For orientation a normal study will be shown (Figure 97 *A, B* and *C*); in figure 97 *A* an anterior view of the abdomen 45 minutes after injection. The liver is well visualized by the ^{131}I rose bengal seen superiorly. No small bowel radio-activity is present yet. The six-hour anterior abdominal view (Figure 97 *B*) shows radioactivity in the duodenum (you can even "see" the ligament of Treitz). By 24 hours radioactivity has passed into the large bowel, as the de-scending colon is seen (Figure 97 *C*).

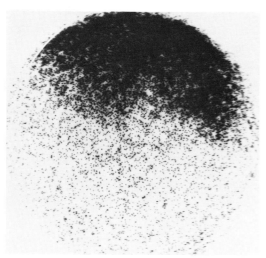

Figure 97 A. Normal anterior rose bengal scan (45 minutes).

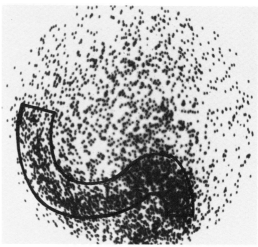

Figure 97 B. Rose bengal scan (upper ab-dominal view, 6 hours).

Figure 97 C. Rose bengal scan (lower abdominal view, 24 hours).

PROBLEM

John Finch, aged four months, is being evaluated for jaundice. This rose bengal scan was obtained and the six- (Figure 97 *D*) and 24-hour (Figure 97 *E*) ante-rior images are shown. Is there any radioactivity in the small bowel? What is the linear structure that appears be-low the inferior border of the liver?

PROBLEM

Aureolin Gamboge, age six weeks, was evaluated for jaundice by this rose bengal study. Is the liver well delineated on the six-hour study (Figure 97 *F*)? Can you identify either large or small bowel on the 24-hour study (Figure 97 *G*)?

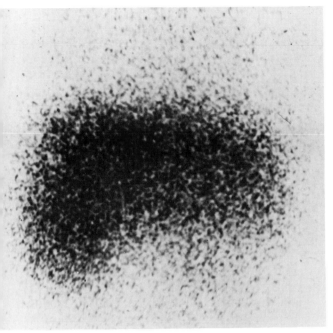

Figure 97 D. *Mr. Finch (6 hours).*

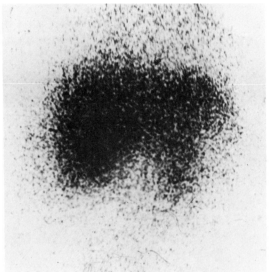

Figure 97 E. *Mr. Finch (24 hours).*

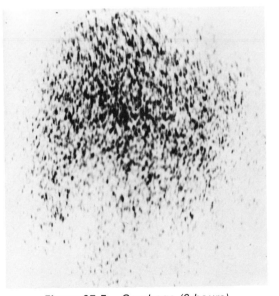

Figure 97 F. *Gamboge (6 hours).*

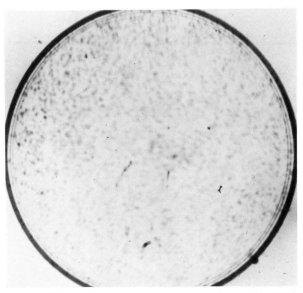

Figure 97 G. *Gamboge (abdominal view, 24 hours).*

(John Finch)

INTERPRETATION: In the six-hour view the liver is well delineated and a suggestion of radioactivity in a structure near the mid-portion of the inferior border is present. By 24 hours the linear structure is well seen and the liver continues to retain radioactivity. This appearance is characteristic of an extra-hepatic biliary obstruction; the linear structure represents the common bile duct.

Diagnosis: At surgery a stenosis of the distal common bile duct was seen. It was probably of congenital origin.

TEACHING POINT: When interpreting the delayed images, the appearance of the liver should be noted as well as any radioactivity seen in the bowel.

Failure of appearance of radio-pharmaceutical in the bowel at 24 hours may be on the basis of obstruction or severe intrinsic liver disease.

(Aureolin Gamboge)

INTERPRETATION: The distribution of radioactivity in the liver image on the six-hour study is irregular. No bowel radioactivity is clearly identified at 24 hours. This combination of images is characteristic of intrinsic liver disease.

Diagnosis: Neonatal hepatitis.

PROBLEM

George Packheaver, a 63 year old man, entered with weight loss, hemoptysis and generalized weakness. His alkaline phosphatase was elevated. *Mr. Packheaver* had a liver scan (Figure 98). How many lesions can you detect? Would you consider multicentric primaries the most likely diagnosis? Before you make your final decision, study *Mr. Packheaver's* chest radiograph.

INTERPRETATION: On the anterior and right lateral views of the liver, multiple focal defects are present. These focal defects, which involve the lateral and inferior aspect of the right lobe of the liver, appear somewhat spherical in their configuration. Analysis of the chest radiograph (Figure 99) gives us a reasonable probability as to the cause of the focal defects within the liver.

Diagnosis: A unilateral hilar mass is present on the left and was found to represent a squamous cell carcinoma. The defects within the liver were metastases.

TEACHING POINT: Multiple lesions of the liver are much more commonly metastases than multiple primaries. Thus, when you encounter several focal defects on a liver scan look elsewhere for the primary.

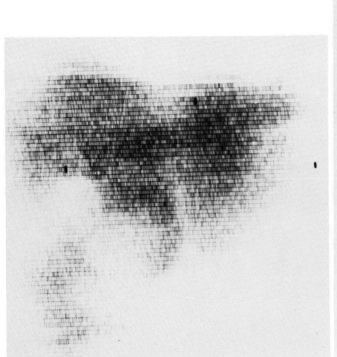

Figure 98 A. *Mr. Packheaver, anterior view, colloid scan.*

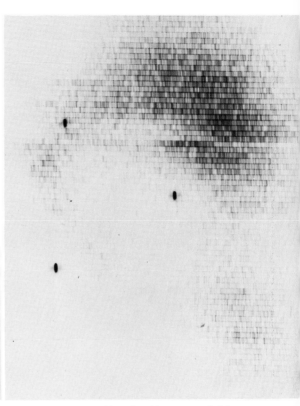

Figure 98 B. *Mr. Packheaver, right lateral view.*

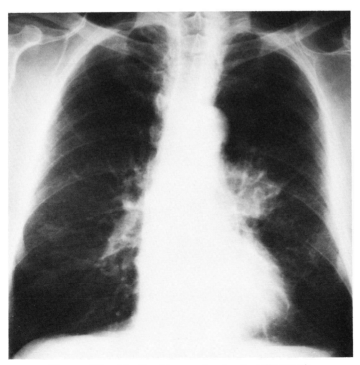

Figure 99. *Mr. Packheaver's chest radiograph.*

PROBLEM

Oscar Throneberry, a 42 year old executive, perforated a chronic duodenal ulcer at a stockholders' meeting. Emergency surgery was performed and the area oversewn. No definitive repair was attempted. Three days following the surgery the patient remained febrile and appeared somewhat septic. The liver profile from blood determinations was distinctly abnormal, and this liver scan was obtained (Figure 100). Again, multiple lesions are seen. Should we now begin a search for a primary neoplasm?

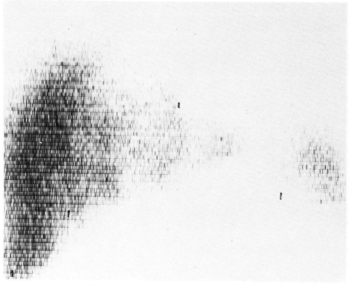

Figure 100. Mr. Throneberry, anterior view, colloid scan.

INTERPRETATION: There is diffusely irregular distribution of radioactivity in the reticuloendothelial system within the medial portion of the right lobe and the entire left lobe of the liver. This has a very similar appearance to the liver scan that one sees with cirrhosis or diffuse metastases, but in this clinical setting was felt most likely to be due to liver inflammation and intrahepatic abscesses. The patient died shortly after the study, and at autopsy there were multiple liver abscesses involving the left lobe and medial portion of the right lobe of the liver.

PROBLEM

Hortense Maltraite is a 43 year old obese female who has had several months of right upper quadrant pain. The gall bladder series revealed nonvisualization of the gall bladder. *Mrs. Maltraite* had a cholecystectomy two weeks ago. Following the operation, she became febrile. An exploratory laparotomy was carried out and revealed an abscess in the area of the gall bladder fossa. Surgical drains were placed and the patient begun on antibiotic therapy. Ten days later the patient continued to be febrile and this liver scan and abdominal radiograph were obtained (Figure 101). The patient has had surgery to this area. Would you expect the defect on the liver scan to be this large?

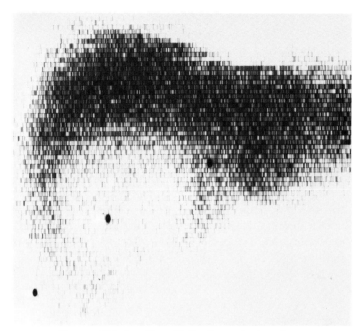

Figure 101 A. *Mrs. Maltraite, anterior view.*

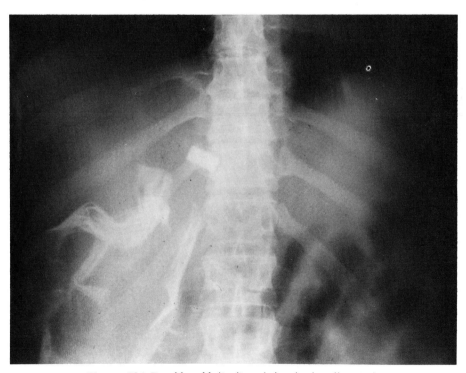

Figure 101 B. *Mrs. Maltraite, abdominal radiograph.*

INTERPRETATION: The defect in radio-activity appears larger than one would anticipate from the operation and placing of a surgical drain. (This is conjectural.) Therefore, it was felt that this probably represented an intrahepatic abscess in the area of the drain. The patient underwent a third operation and an abscess *was* found in this area of the liver.

Diagnosis: Intrahepatic abscess.

TEACHING POINT: You should be as critical about attributing postoperative lesions to surgical manifestations as you are to normal variations. The size, location and configuration of structures should be predictable from the knowledge you have of the surgery.

PROBLEM
Hanah Sofine, 63, had an esophageal diverticulum and chronic aspiration pneumonia. An intravenous catheter monitor was placed in the superior vena cava. Unfortunately *Mrs. Sofine* had an overwhelming *Candida albicans* septicemia and developed a lung abscess (detected on the chest radiograph). Because of abnormal liver chemistry values, she had a liver scan (Figure 102). Is this a prominent porta?

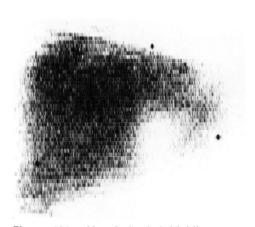

Figure 102. *Mrs. Sofine's initial liver scan.*

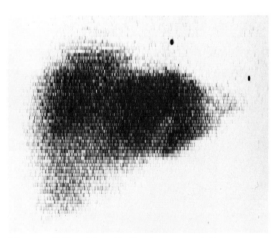

Figure 103. *Mrs. Sofine's second liver scan, two weeks later.*

INTERPRETATION: There is a defect within the medial portion of the right lobe of the liver. (Minimal irregularity is seen within the entire right lower border. This was felt to be normal anatomical thinning of liver parenchyma).

The patient was placed on amphotericin B therapy. Two weeks later she was remarkably improved. A subsequent liver scan was obtained (Figure 103). Do you notice any improvement? There is return of the reticuloendothelial function within the medial part of the right lobe. Only a small defect is now noted.

Diagnosis: Abscess due to fungus disease; treated; with improvement.

PROBLEM

Clara Shipwright, a 43 year old woman, had an abnormal BSP retention of 13 per cent. Her anterior and right lateral liver scans are also interesting (Figure 104 A and B). An extensive diagnostic eval- uation failed to reveal a primary neo- plasm. The patient appeared in good health, was afebrile and was not in the least interested in having hepatic angiography.

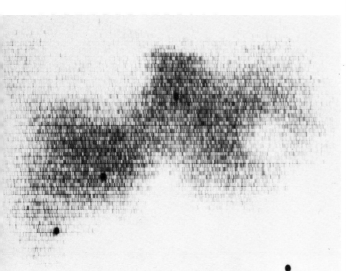

Figure 104 A. *Mrs. Shipwright (sulfur colloid scan). (From DeLand, F. H., and Wagner, H. N.:* Atlas of Nu- clear Medicine, *Vol. 3, 1972.)*

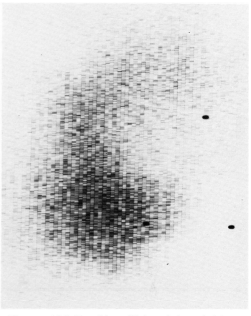

Figure 104 B. *Mrs. Shipwright, right lateral view.*

INTERPRETATION: Two large defects are seen on the liver scan in the superior aspect of the right lobe and the left lobe of the liver. These lesions were thought to be either multiple neoplasms of the liver or (more likely) metastases.

Physical examination revealed wide- spread telangiectasia. On the remote possibility that this might represent in- trahepatic hemangiomas, a scan was performed using an intravascular blood pool agent (^{113}In-labeled transferrin) (Figure 105 A and B).

If the lesions are vascular, the de- fects should disappear. However, one could be misled by a necrotic center in a lesion of any type. Vascular hepatomas and sarcomas, in the limited experience that we are aware of, remain as defects on the scan with intravascular agents.

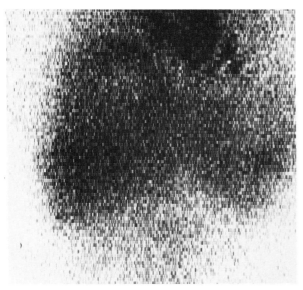

Figure 105 A. *Liver blood-pool scan, anterior view. (From DeLand, F. H., and Wagner, H. N.: Atlas of Nuclear Medicine, Vol. 3, 1972.)*

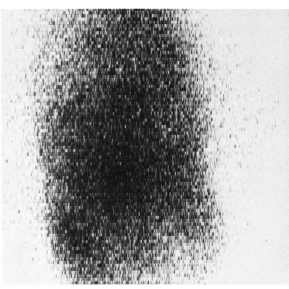

Figure 105 B. *Liver blood-pool scan, right lateral view.*

INTERPRETATION: The anterior and lateral views show that the lesions present on the previous scan are now "filled in" by the intravascular agent. (On the anterior view the dense radioactivity superiorly is within the cardiac chamber).

An open biopsy was obtained. The pathological diagnosis was hemangioma.

Diagnosis: Multiple congenital hemangiomas of the liver.

SPLEEN SCANNING

Imaging of the spleen by either injection of a colloidal substance or utilization of labeled red blood cells in which the surface has been altered or damaged affords an innocuous method of visualizing this organ.

Labeling of red blood cells with sodium chromate (^{51}Cr), mercury mercurihydroxypropane (^{197}Hg) or ^{99m}Tc are reliable methods that have proved clinically useful. The spleen is seen as an ovoid area of radioactivity that is normally oriented obliquely in the left upper quadrant. This distribution of radioactivity is uniform (Figure 106 A and B).

In many disease states affecting the liver, the spleen will become enlarged (Figure 106 C). Therefore, the area of radioactivity on the spleen scan will appear much larger than is normally seen. Because of its varied orientation within the left upper quadrant, splenic enlargement should be visualized in more than one projection before it is considered a definitely abnormal finding.

It has been our experience that when the spleen enlarges it does not do so in an absolutely homogeneous manner, and the distribution of radioactivity may appear somewhat irregular (Figure 106 D). This is especially true if the enlargement is due to infiltrative disease. However, large focal areas of diminished activity should not be present. This probably reflects that the trapping of damaged RBC's is not absolutely uniform throughout the gland.

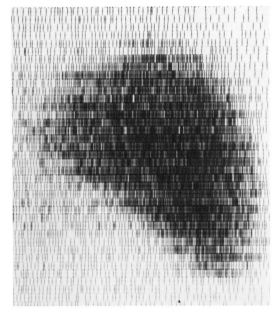

Figure 106 A. *Spleen (normal anterior view).*

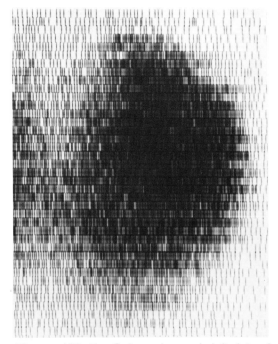

Figure 106 B. *Spleen (normal left lateral view).*

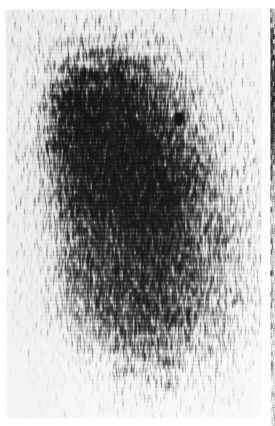

Figure 106 C. *Splenomegaly, anterior view.*

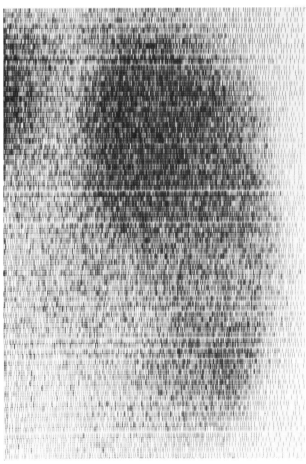

Figure 106 D. *Splenomegaly, anterior view.*

PROBLEM

Reid Sternburg, 27, has noted decreased exercise tolerance, weight loss and generalized myalgia for the past several months. On physical examination, multiple nodes were palpated in his neck and axilla. This scan was obtained with ^{99m}Tc (technetium) sulfur colloid as the radiopharmaceutical (Figure 107). Both the liver and spleen are visualized. What is your opinion regarding the size of the left lobe of the liver and the spleen?

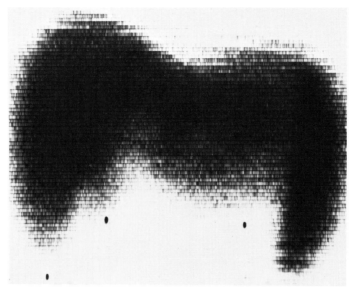

Figure 107. Reid Sternburg, anterior view.

INTERPRETATION: Both hepato- and splenomegaly are present, with the spleen markedly enlarged. Because of the patient's age and generalized symptoms, the diagnosis of Hodgkin's disease was suggested. This was confirmed by cervical node biopsy. Both hepatic and splenic involvement were later proved at exploratory laparotomy.

TEACHING POINT: Reticuloendothelial scanning has been utilized in staging of malignant disease. When the spleen is affected with lymphoma it may show enlargement, focal abnormalities, or appear normal.

The next patient, **Lavender Herring,** has known reticulum cell sarcoma. Only an anterior view of her colloid scan (^{99m}Tc sulfur colloid) is shown because this strikingly abnormal image was *only* seen in this view (Figure 108). Could you explain the abnormality from the concomitant abdominal radiograph (Figure 109)?

INTERPRETATION: A large focal defect is present in the anterior view of the spleen image. However, the patient had a barium enema the previous day and the gamma rays (140 KEV from ^{99m}Tc) were shielded from the detector by the barium in the splenic flexure. This "defect" is an artifact (maybe even a red herring).

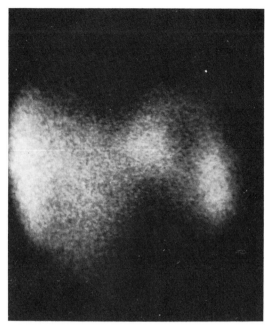

Figure 108. Miss Herring, anterior view of spleen (camera view on Polaroid film, spleen and liver are "white"). (Courtesy of Dr. Magic Potsaid.)

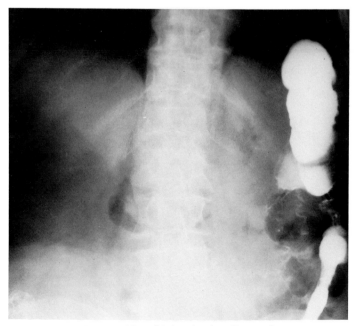

Figure 109. Abdominal radiograph.

PROBLEM

Red Johnson, 66, is seen because of anemia. On physical examination, the spleen was enlarged to palpation. Radiographs of the bone showed increased density with an increased trabecular pattern. A spleen scan was obtained with ^{197}Hg BMHP, which goes only to the spleen (Figure 110 A and B, anterior and left lateral).

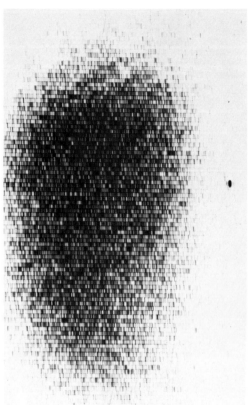

Figure 110 A. *Red Johnson, anterior spleen scan.*

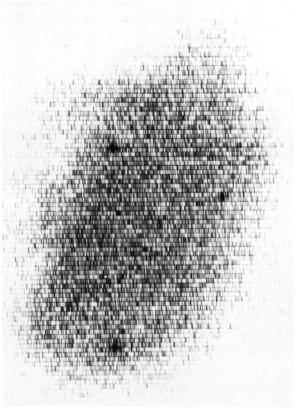

Figure 110 B. *Red Johnson, left lateral spleen scan.*

INTERPRETATION: There is gross splenomegaly, with irregular uptake of the radiopharmaceutical within the spleen. The clinical picture, the radiographic findings and the enlarged spleen on the scan are most consistent with the diagnosis of Hodgkin's disease. However, a biopsy of enlarged nodes showed chronic inflammatory changes. The patient's skin test for histoplasmosis was positive. Removal of the patient's spleen for staging of his "lymphoma" revealed that he had generalized histoplasmosis.

PROBLEM

Gregory Eisenmenger, 24, is anemic and has a holosystolic murmur along the left sternal border. He is being evaluated for these findings. Because of an episode of acute left upper quadrant pain, a spleen scan (Figure 111 A, anterior view scintillation camera) was obtained after barium gastrointestinal studies were negative. What is the distribution of radioactivity in the spleen? Can the clinical presentation and the scan abnormalities be related?

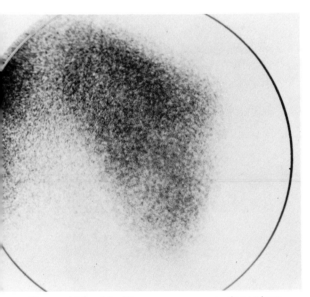

Figure 111. Mr. Eisenmenger, anterior spleen scan.

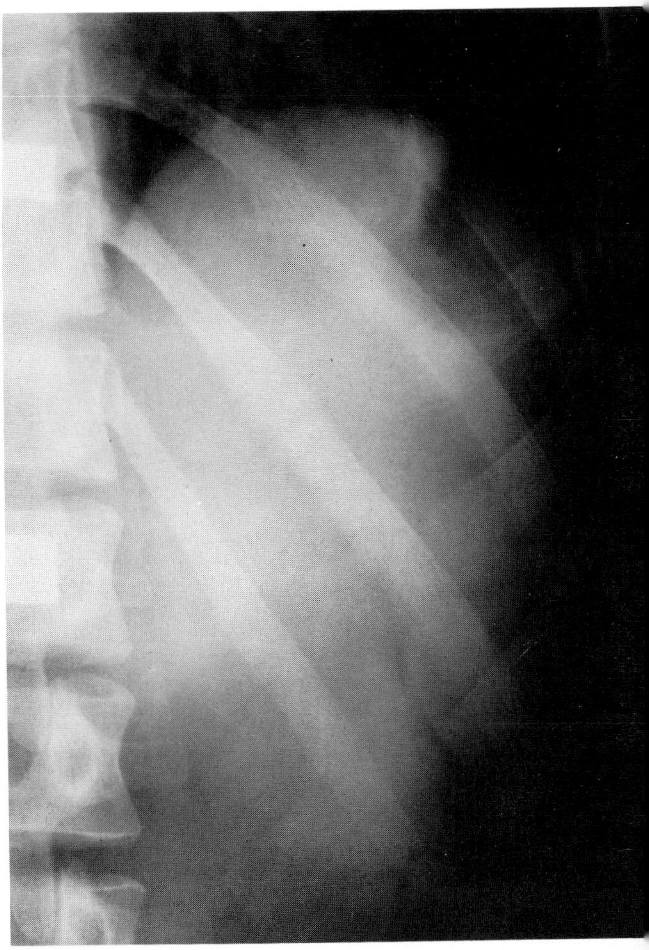

Figure 112. Abdominal radiograph (ignore technical defect over diaphragm laterally).

INTERPRETATION: There is irregular radiopharmaceutical distribution within the enlarged spleen. On the abdominal radiograph there is confirmation of the splenomegaly (Figure 112).

Diagnosis: This patient had a ventricular septal defect and subacute bacterial endocarditis. An enlarged spleen is often associated with this disorder, and the irregular defects within the spleen probably represent small septic emboli.

PROBLEM

Brooks Flank, 17, presents with severe abdominal pain. After approximately six hours, the diffuse pain became localized to the left upper quadrant. *Mr. Flank* had a spleen scan, obtained with ^{197}Hg BMHP-labeled red blood cells (Figure 113, anterior view). Can you identify the boundaries of the spleen?

INTERPRETATION: There is almost no radioactivity within the spleen. This appearance would suggest that almost no splenic function is present. Within several days the patient's symptoms decreased and he was discharged from the hospital. He returned on an outpatient basis three months later, and a repeat spleen scan was obtained (Figure 114, anterior view). The appearance of this image is quite different from the previous scan. Could you describe the difference in functional terms?

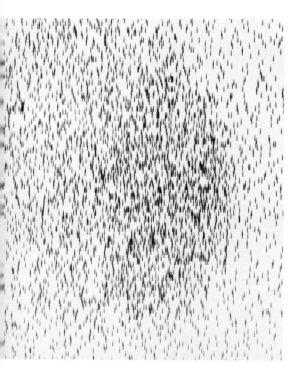

Figure 113. *Initial spleen scan.*

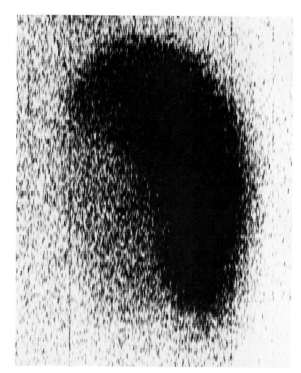

Figure 114. *Spleen scan three months later.*

ANALYSIS: The spleen scan appears much more normal, although the spleen is slightly enlarged. Such a dramatic difference between the two spleen scans suggests that the acute episode temporarily eliminated spleen function, but no residual diminished function is present. Careful attention to the selected bone radiographs will allow a definitive diagnosis (Figure 115 A and B). The bones of the pelvis appear somewhat dense and show a coarsened trabecular pattern. Diminished vertebral height, which appears to affect the mid-portion of the vertebrae, is present. This decrease in height occurs within each vertebrae in the central area. These are findings characteristic of those seen in sickle cell anemia.

Diagnosis: Sickle cell anemia with abdominal crisis causing diminished spleen function during the acute episode.

TEACHING POINT: This series of events has been reported in patients with sickle cell anemia and is felt to be due to sludging of the abnormal cells within the spleen. Gradual congestion of the spleen occurs until the organ is so filled with the abnormal red blood cells that it becomes temporarily functionless. Following the acute episode the abnormal cells are gradually eliminated from the spleen and normal function is restored.

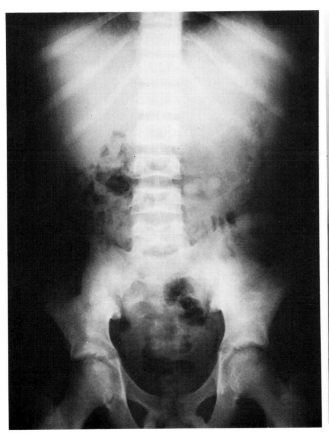

Figure 115 A. Abdominal radiograph.

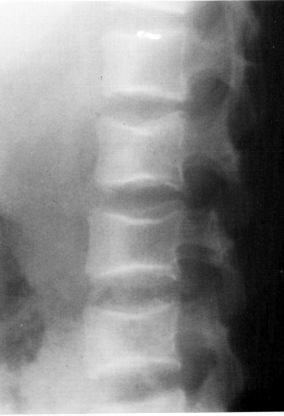

Figure 115 B. Lumbar spine radiograph.

PANCREATIC IMAGING

The ability to image the pancreas selectively is a goal that has long been sought but has not been entirely achieved. Imaging of this organ depends upon the accumulation of a radioactively labeled precursor of amino acids. Selenium-75 is incorporated into the structure of methionine as a substitute for the sulfur atom. This forms selenium-75 selenomethionine. Because amino acid production in the pancreas is rapid, within minutes after intravenous injection, the radiopharmaceutical will be localized to the pancreatic area. However, there is much amino acid production in the liver, a larger organ, and radioactivity there will often be seen overlying the pancreatic image (Figure 116, drawing). Many methods have been proposed to remove the liver image from the field of view by positioning, or by labeling the liver with another radiopharmaceutical of different photon energy and electronically subtracting the liver image from that of the pancreas.

You will see lesions in the pancreas as areas of either focal or generalized decrease in radioactivity. Neoplasms and inflammatory lesions of the pancreas do not have characteristic features to distinguish them from each other. Both false negative and false positive studies have been reported. At present,

pancreatic scanning is probably an insensitive screening procedure. If the pancreatic scan is normal and the pancreas is visualized in its entirety, there is *probably* no pancreatic disease present. If an abnormal scan is obtained, then this may represent nonvisualization of the pancreas for technical reasons, an unexplained normal variant, inflammation or malignancy.

The three figures on the opposite page represent three normal studies of the pancreas. These studies were made 2 to 60 minutes after intravenous injection of 150 to 250 μCi of ^{75}Se selenomethionine. A scintillation camera was utilized as the imaging device. The first study (Figure 117) was made with the camera placed upon the abdomen of a patient lying supine. The next two figures (Figures 118 and 119) were made from the anterior aspect also, but with the patient turned in various degrees of obliquity toward the right side. This maneuver is helpful in separating the pancreas from the liver.

The liver is the dense area of radioactivity in the upper left quadrant of the figure (the patient's right upper quadrant). The shape of the pancreas is variable and has been described in such terms as "banana or boomerang" in configuration. The major criterion for recognizing a normal pancreas is not its shape but whether or not the distribution of radioactivity in the organ is reasonably homogeneous.

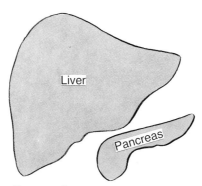

Figure 116. *Pancreatic scan with ^{75}Se (selenomethionine).*

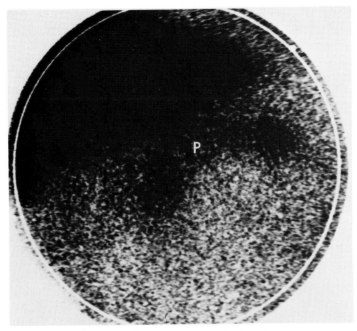

Figure 117. *Pancreas, anterior view.*

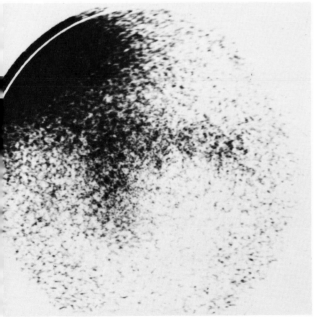

Figure 118. *Pancreas, anterior oblique view.*

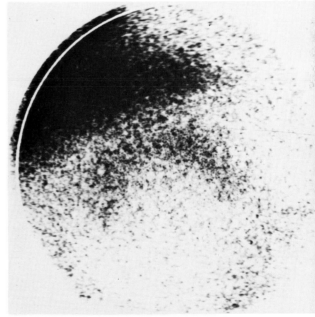

Figure 119. *Pancreas, anterior oblique view.*

Samuel Rumpus was in excellent health until three months prior to admission, when he gradually began having back pain that did not respond to "manipulation." He has lost 27 pounds and has noted general fatigue and decreasing appetite. A pancreatic scan (Figure 120) was obtained after his gastrointestinal series was normal. Can you outline the entire pancreas? [If you can, *go directly to Jail!*]

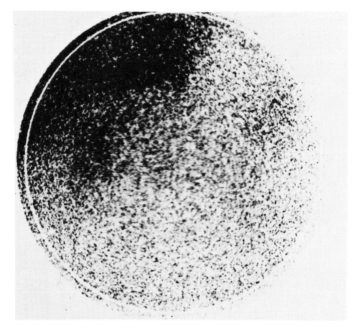

Figure 120. *Samuel Rumpus' pancreatic scan (anterior view).*

INTERPRETATION: The radioactivity superiorly is in the liver. Just below, a small oblong collection of radioactivity is seen which represents the head of the pancreas. The midportion does not appear to contain radioactivity, but there is an accumulation to the patient's left, thought to represent the tail. This image was interpreted as a focal abnormality of the mid-portion of the pancreas.

Diagnosis: At surgery a large carcinoma of the mid-pancreas *was* present.

Smash Pickle, 36, enters the emergency room for the tenth time because of acute abdominal pain. According to the patient, he had sudden, severe mid-epigastric pain several hours prior to admission while attending a party. Several members of his entourage say that the pain could not have been anything

Smash had eaten because he had been on "a liquid diet" for quite some time. This abdominal radiograph (Figure 121) and pancreatic scan were obtained (Figure 122). Can you correlate the calcific densities, clinical history and scan findings?

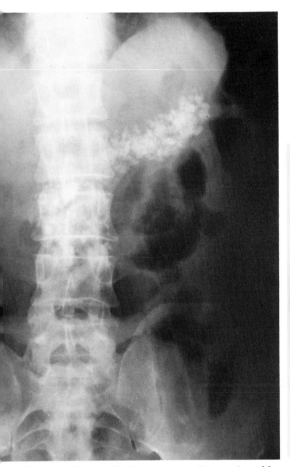

Figure 121. Abdominal radiograph, Mr. Pickle (plain film).

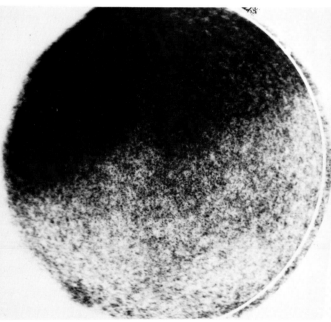

Figure 122. Smash Pickle, anterior pancreatic scan.

INTERPRETATION: On the abdominal radiograph you can see diffuse calcification in the pancreatic area. His pancreas is poorly visualized with the selenium-75 selenomethionine scan. The presumptive diagnosis of acute pancreatitis was confirmed by the elevated serum amylase, a left pleural effusion and the patient's subsequent clinical course.

TEACHING POINT: As you have seen from the above examples pancreatic scanning is a relatively insensitive nonspecific procedure.

CHAPTER IV

KIDNEY

RENAL IMAGING

From the previous "Exercises" you know that radiopaque contrast medium is handled in a dynamic fashion by the kidneys. The accumulation, transit and subsequent concentration of the iodinated contrast within the collecting system of the urinary tract is familiar to you. Some radiopharmaceuticals pass through the kidney after intravenous injection in much the same manner, producing "dynamic" images.

On the other hand, the mercurial agents are both excreted *and* concentrated by the tubules, thus visualizing the functioning renal parenchyma. Approximately 80 per cent of mercury neohydrin is excreted within 24 hours, while 20 per cent is retained in the proximal renal tubules. Therefore, these compounds are suitable radiopharmaceuticals for "static" images of the kidneys (Figure 123 A).

A more dynamic analysis of renal function can be obtained by a substance which is visualized in the vascular phase of its delivery to the kidney (Figure 123 B) in its transit through the renal substance (Figure 123 C) and, finally, in its concentration in the renal collecting systems as it passes to the urinary bladder (Figure 123 D). A number of radiopharmaceuticals have been developed which, in varying degrees, act as glomerular substances (are cleared by glomerular filtration) and have the property of allowing dynamic structural images. These are true glomerular substances and are excreted by the kidney much the same as inulin. Examples are chelates, such as diethylene-triamine-penta-acetic acid (DTPA).

The patient is positioned either prone or supine in front of a scintillation camera for the dynamic imaging. A large intravenous bolus of radioactivity (approximately 10 to 15 mCi) usually is injected, and multiple views are obtained at five-second intervals through the vascular and early parenchymal phases (Figure 124). After the excretory phase is reached, in which there is visualization of the radioactivity within the renal pelvis and collecting systems, views are obtained at five- to 10-minute intervals until radioactivity is present within the bladder (Figure 124, lower row).

This dynamic study may be performed at the same time as a static study with a tubular agent, if the photon energy is sufficiently different. From this method you can obtain structural detail as well as a dynamic expression of renal physiology.

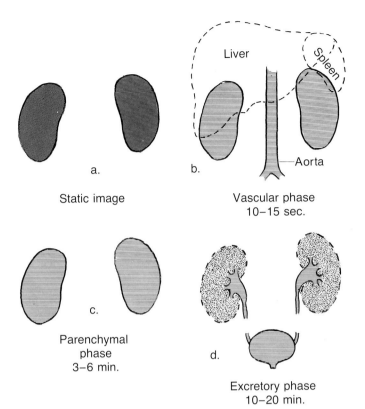

Figure 123. *Dynamic renal image (anterior view).* ^{197}*Hg used in* (a). ^{99}*Tc DTPA (chelate) used in* (b), (c) *and* (d).

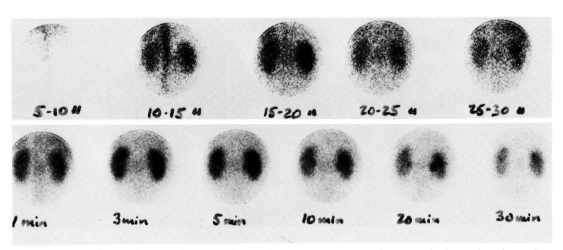

Figure 124. *Normal dynamic image (posterior view; upper row in seconds, lower in minutes).*

INTERPRETATION OF THE RENAL SCAN

On the dynamic renal image (obtained with a radiopharmaceutical such as ^{99m}Tc DTPA, a chelate) the early portion of the vascular phase should show radioactivity within the abdominal aorta (Figure 124, 10 to 15 seconds). This is represented by a band of radioactivity running vertically in the mid-line. The renal arteries are not seen. Several seconds later, the renal parenchyma will be visualized as paired concentrations of radioactivity (Figure 125, enlarged camera view). Any disparity between the onset of visualization of one kidney in comparison with the other in the early phases should be analyzed in the later phases of the dynamic views for delayed excretion. Radioactivity will normally leave the abdominal aorta and appear to accumulate in the renal substance itself. During the transit phase, the size and shape as well as position of the kidneys can be assessed (Figure 125). The renal pelvis and collecting structures will then be visualized as concavities in the medial surface of the radioactivity in the renal parenchyma. When the excretory phase is reached, this concavity will fill with radioactivity and present as a medial convexity (Figure 126). As the radiopharmaceutical passes through the glomeruli and concentrates in the collecting system, the renal parenchyma will appear to become smaller. The rate of decrease of the radioactivity within the renal parenchyma has been referred to as the "renal transit time."

The ureters are not usually visualized but, if so, are seen only faintly (Figure 127). Total visualization of the ureter as a linear structure passing from the pelvis to the bladder is seen in patients with severe hydroureter and vesicoureteral reflux. The urinary bladder appears much the same as on intravenous urography, a spherical concentration in the suprapubic region.

Vesicoureteral reflux may be detected by instillation of a radiopharmaceutical into the bladder through a catheter and imaging of the abdomen during voiding. Radioactivity passing

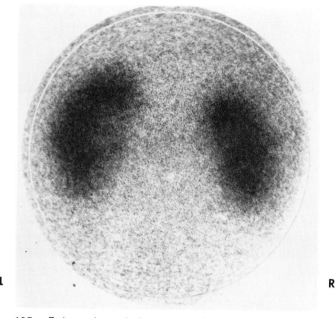

L   R

Figure 125. *Enlarged renal view, parenchymal phase (posterior view).*

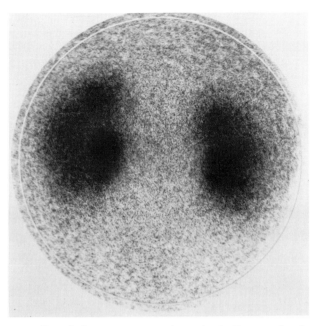

Figure 126. Renal view, excretory phase (note the renal pelves here).

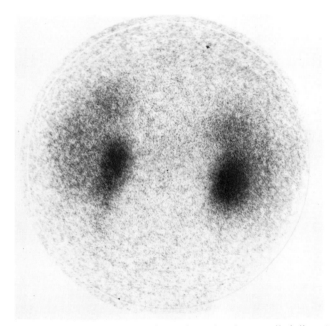

Figure 127. Late excretory phase (renal pelves well delineated).

up the ureters (reflux) will then be identified. Quantification of the dynamic study by any method of computation and image analysis will probably increase the amount of information de- rived from these studies. A small computer coupled with a display format and a method of selective area analysis is employed in many laboratories.

PROBLEM

George Grawitz, 58, presented with a right abdominal mass and hematuria. *Mr. Grawitz* had a dynamic scan of his kidneys (Figure 128). Images from the early vascular phase, late vascular phase and parenchymal phase (Figure 128 A, B and C) are shown. Can you identify and characterize the right abdominal mass?

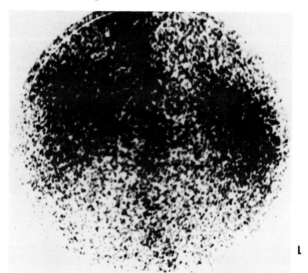

R   L

Figure 128 A. Mr. Grawitz: Dynamic renal image, vascular phase (anterior view).

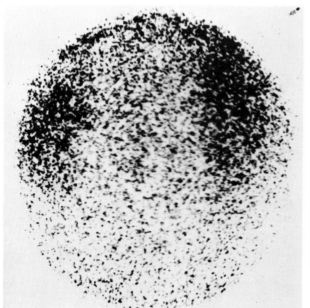

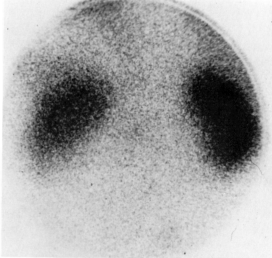

Figure 128 C. Dynamic renal image, parenchymal phase.

Figure 128 B. Dynamic renal image, late vascular phase.

INTERPRETATION: In the early vascular phase the blood pools appear approximately equal. The later phases of the dynamic study show diminished transit of the radiopharmaceutical in the right kidney. The differences between the lower poles are greater than the upper.

This would suggest a lesion in the right lower pole which might represent a cyst, or neoplastic invasion.

His nephrotomogram (Figure 129) and renal angiogram (Figure 130) will allow you to make a specific diagnosis.

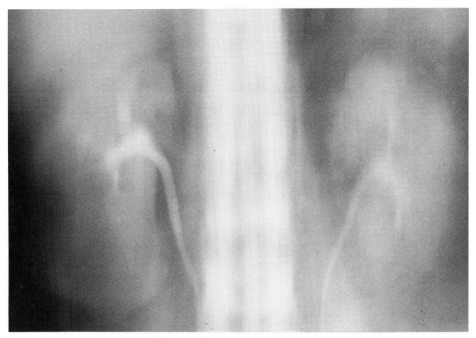

Figure 129. *Nephrotomogram.*

Diagnosis: The right lower pole mass is seen. It appears solid because it has the same radiographic density as the rest of the kidney and distorts the lower pole collecting system. Irregular, abnormal vessels are present in the selective renal angiogram and supply the lower pole mass. Hypertrophied capsular vessels supplying the lesion are present inferiorly. These abnormal vessels are diagnostic of a renal cell carcinoma.

TEACHING POINT: Renal neoplasms usually appear as areas of diminished radioactivity in the parenchymal phase, and only occasionally show normal or increased radioactivity in the early vascular phase. The appearance in the vascular phase probably corresponds to the many abnormal vessels present on angiograms.

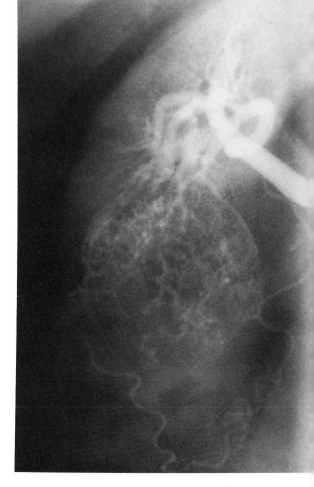

Figure 130. *Renal angiogram.*

PROBLEM

Bruce Wheeler, 59, enters the hospital with acute renal failure and a blood urea nitrogen of 130. On intravenous urography there was nonvisualization of the kidneys. A retrograde pyelogram showed no evidence of urinary tract obstruction. A static renal scan was obtained with ^{197}Hg mercury chlormerodin (Figure 131). Can you identify any functioning renal parenchyma?

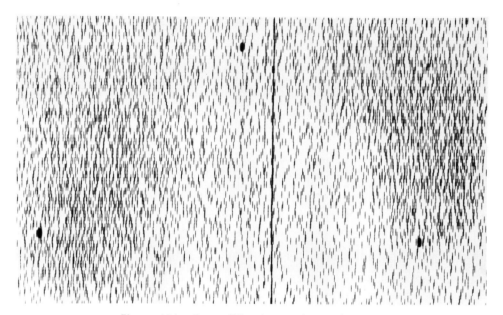

Figure 131. *Bruce Wheeler, static renal scan.*

INTERPRETATION: *Mr. Wheeler's* history was at least suggestive of a vascular lesion, and appropriate studies were obtained.

There is faint visualization of both renal structures, which appear somewhat enlarged but are difficult to outline. The abdominal angiogram (Figure 132) shows delayed renal vascular filling and slow circulation, with separation of the intrarenal arteries. This finding suggests edema of the kidneys bilaterally.

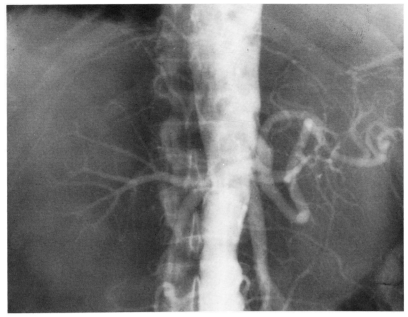

Figure 132. Mr. Wheeler's abdominal angiogram.

An inferior vena cavagram (Figure 133) demonstrates massive bilateral renal vein reflux of contrast material, which is indicative of absence of blood flow from the renal veins. No definite intravenous clots or filling defects are noted. These findings could be caused by a number of acute renal diseases, but in this patient are more suggestive of peripheral renal vein thrombosis.

Final Diagnosis: Bilateral peripheral renal vein thrombosis.

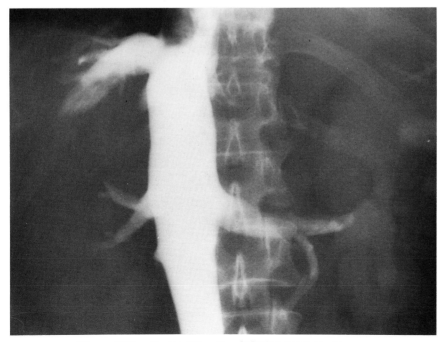

Figure 133. Bruce Wheeler, inferior vena cavagram.

PROBLEM

Blake Star, 43, enters with right flank pain of abrupt onset. An intravenous urogram showed poor renal function on the left side with no visualization on the right. A scan with mercury-197 chlormerodin was obtained (Figure 134). Does the scan abnormality agree with the urogram findings?

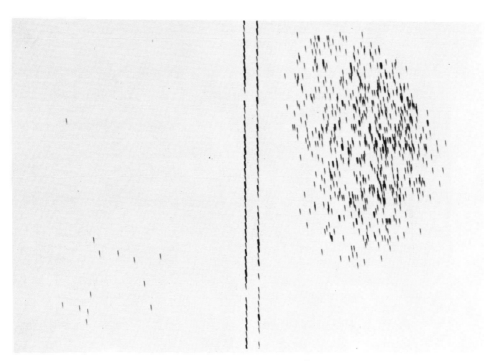

Figure 134. Blake Star, static scan.

INTERPRETATION: The static image shows diffuse irregular uptake of radionuclide in the left kidney with nonvisualization of the right kidney. The important question is whether or not there is a right kidney present. This can be answered by the abdominal radiograph (Figure 135).

The abdominal radiograph shows that there is, indeed, a right renal structure present. The chest radiograph may allow us to properly understand the patient's clinical history (Figure 136 *A* and *B*).

On his chest radiograph there is evidence of a sterniotomy incision, with metallic sutures and a prosthetic valve in the aortic area. *Mr. Star* had clinical manifestations of multiple emboli and undoubtedly had a major embolus to the right renal artery. Smaller emboli were probably the cause for the diffuse irregularity of radiopharmaceutical distribution in the left renal area.

Diagnosis: Renal artery embolus.

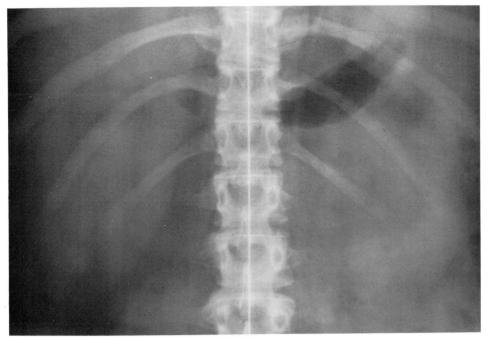

Figure 135. Abdominal radiograph.

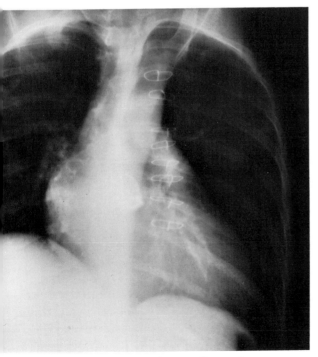

Figure 136 A. Star's chest radiograph.

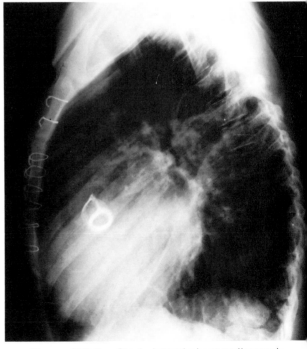

Figure 136 B. Star's lateral chest radiograph.

PROBLEM

Gloria E. Finchley, 32, was in an automobile accident and sustained trauma to her left side. She entered the hospital with left flank pain and hematuria. An intravenous urogram was reported as normal. However, the outline of the renal parenchyma in the left lower pole was not so well delineated as the right. She had a static renal scan (Figure 137). Compare the size of the right and left kidneys. Can you decide if any part of a kidney does not contain radioactivity?

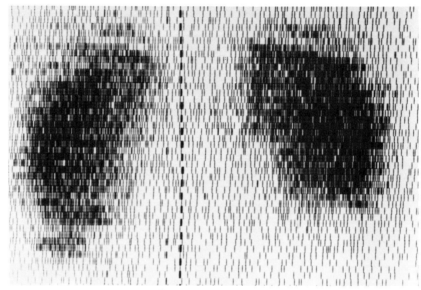

Figure 137. Gloria Finchley, static renal scan.

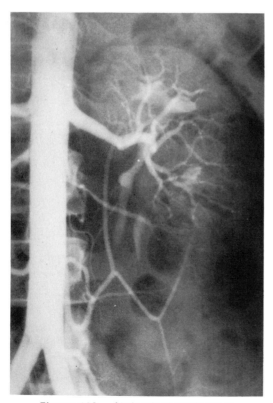

Figure 138. Abdominal angiogram.

INTERPRETATION: The left lower pole of the renal parenchyma does not accumulate radiopharmaceutical. (There is some irregularity in the extreme upper and lower pole of the kidneys bilaterally due to patient motion; however, the findings within the left lower pole were felt to be significant and not due to motion.) An abdominal angiogram (Figure 138) was obtained and shows filling and good perfusion of the upper and mid-portions of the left kidney. The lower pole of the left kidney is supplied by an accessory renal artery (originating approximately one vertebral width below the main renal artery), which is very irregular in its contour.

At operation there was bleeding in the wall of this accessory renal artery and compromise of the lumen. An infarction of the left lower pole supplied by this artery was present.

Diagnosis: Trauma to the accessory renal artery which supplied the left lower pole.

PROBLEM

Annie Gurley Smith, 33, enters the hospital for evaluation of recent onset of hypertension. She had a renal scan with mercury-197 chlormerodin (Figure 139). Are the abnormalities unilateral or bilateral?

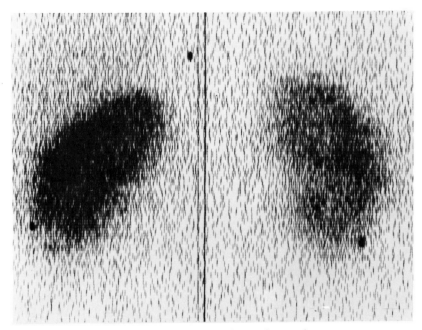

Figure 139. *Miss Smith, static renal scan.*

INTERPRETATION: Diffuse irregularity of radiopharmaceutical distribution is present in the left kidney. The right kidney appears normal. The scan would suggest that some unilateral process involves *Miss Smith's* kidney. An angiogram was obtained (Figure 140). In the abdominal angiogram, irregularity and "beading" of both renal vessels are seen. This is characteristic of renal artery dysplasia (fibromuscular hyperplasia) and appears to affect both her kidneys equally. Therefore, the scan findings and the angiographic abnormalities do not seem to correlate in this case.

Diagnosis: Renal artery dysplasia.

TEACHING POINT: Dynamic and static renal imaging is useful as a screening test for unilateral renal hypertension. Although both false positives and negatives are encountered, this type of study is probably more sensitive than the intravenous urogram.

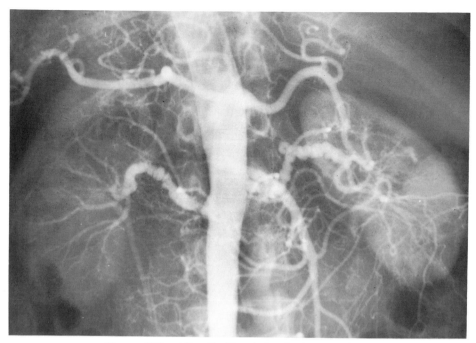

Figure 140. Miss Smith, abdominal angiogram.

PROBLEM

Constance Manley is a 28 year old hypertensive "spokesman" for women's lib. Because of the patient's hypertension, this static renal scan was obtained (Figure 141).

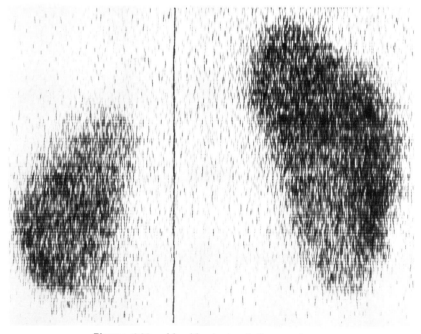

Figure 141. Ms. Manley's static renal scan.

INTERPRETATION: The left kidney is large, and a diffuse irregular distribution of activity is seen within it. The right kidney is either small or some areas of the renal parenchyma do not accumulate the ^{197}Hg chlormerodin. Her liver scan may give some insight into this patient's condition (Figure 142).

Multiple focal defects within the liver parenchyma are present and appear to involve both the right and left lobes. With multiple defects of both kidneys and the liver, certain congenital disorders come to mind! A glance at the capillary phase of the abdominal angiogram (Figure 143) will allow a definite diagnosis in this case.

Diagnosis: This patient had congenital polycystic disease affecting both the liver and the kidneys.

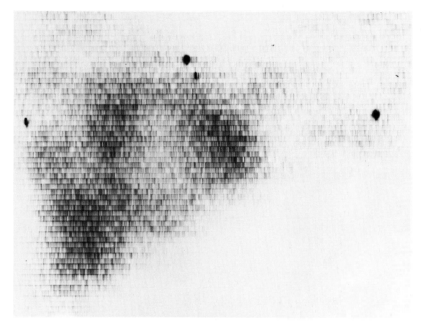

Figure 142. Ms. Manley's liver scan, anterior.

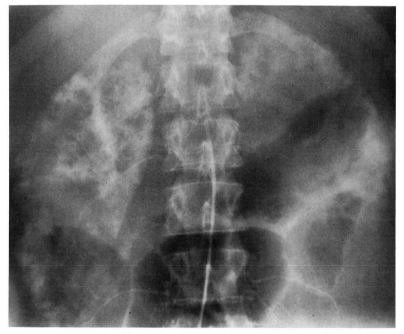

Figure 143. Ms. Manley's abdominal angiogram, capillary phase.

PROBLEM

Atlas Buffaloe, 9, is being evaluated for urinary urgency and frequency. This dynamic renal scan was obtained in the prone position; thus, the patient's right side is to your right. The parenchymal phase from five minutes to 20 minutes after injection is shown (Figure 144). Is the transit through the left kidney slow? (Compare with bottom row, Figure 124.) What do you think the lobulated collection of radioactivity represents? A single view of the intravenous urogram at 30 minutes oriented in the same manner should prove most helpful (Figure 145).

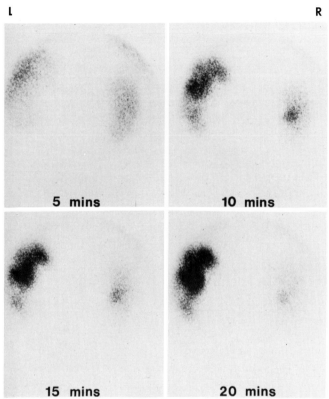

Figure 144. *Atlas Buffaloe, dynamic renal scan with patient prone.*

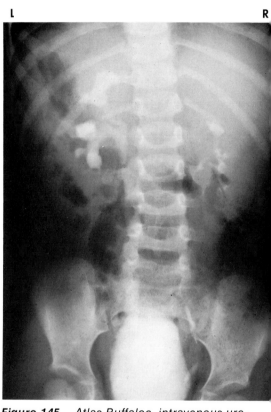

Figure 145. *Atlas Buffaloe, intravenous urogram.*

INTERPRETATION: Lobulated structures that fill late in the parenchymal phase and concentrate radioactivity most likely represent dilated calyces. The intravenous urogram (Figure 145) shows dilated and "blunted" calyces on the left side with minimal changes on the right. *Atlas* had an acute pyelonephritis with caliectasis, hydronephrosis and hydroureter.

TEACHING POINT: The dynamic renal scan may contain enough structural detail to delineate dilated collecting structures in patients with caliectasis, hydronephrosis and hydroureter. Delayed studies must be obtained to visualize the ureters. When dilatation has been present for several months as a result of obstruction or severe reflux, the renal function may be so severely damaged that these structures will not be seen on an intravenous urogram. They often will visualize on a dynamic renal scan, however.

PROBLEM

Finnigan Frock, 6, has one of the severe forms of spinal dysrhaphia, consisting of absence of the sacrum and coccyx. Because of attendant urinary problems this dynamic renal scan was obtained (Figure 146 *A*). The parenchymal phase from one to 25 minutes is shown. Are the bladder and ureters seen in these images (made with the patient in the supine position)? Figure 146 *B* is a view from a voiding cystogram and contains greater structural information, allowing you to arrive at a reasonable explanation for the scan findings.

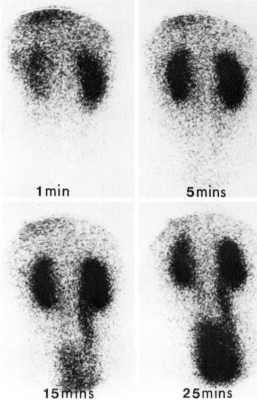

Figure 146 A. *Finnigan Frock, dynamic renal image (anterior view).*

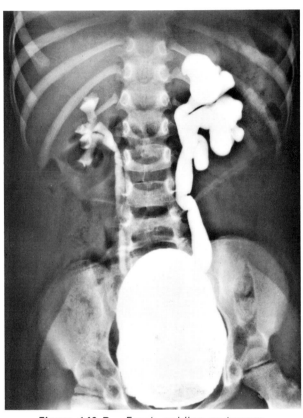

Figure 146 B. *Frock, voiding cystogram.*

INTERPRETATION: Radioactivity is present in both renal areas during the early parenchymal phase of the scan. The right side contains much less radioactivity initially than the left, but by 15 minutes the collecting structures are well seen. The left ureter is clearly defined passing to an enlarged bladder. A linear area of radioactivity leading from the right kidney to the bladder probably represents the right ureter but is not well delineated. It may be that by 25 minutes accumulation of the radiopharmaceutical in the right kidney has not been sufficient to pass into and adequately visualize the ureter. From this study you should suspect hydronephrosis and hydroureter bilaterally.

The voiding cystourethrogram shows marked bilateral reflux from a large irregular bladder. Hydronephrosis and hydroureter are present bilaterally but are much more marked on the left.

Diagnosis: Neurogenic bladder with vesicoureteral reflux, hydronephrosis and hydroureter.

CHAPTER V

BONE AND BONE MARROW

BONE AND BONE MARROW SCANNING

The accumulation of any radiopharmaceutical utilized for bone scanning in a particular osseous area is dependent upon the blood flow, the amount of extracellular space and the metabolic activity. Several of the radiopharmaceuticals employed exchange with calcium in the osseous matrix. Others exchange with hydroxyl groups in the hydroxyapatite crystal or in various elements within the ground substance of the bone.

Any abnormality of bone which causes an increased metabolic turnover or blood flow will be reflected as an area of increased radiopharmaceutical accumulation. *Therefore, both benign and malignant lesions may be seen as abnormal areas of radiopharmaceutical concentration.* Neoplasms and inflammatory conditions will often cause localized increases in radiopharmaceutical and are, thus, indistinguishable from each other. Lytic lesions within the bone probably do not have predominantly osteoblastic activity in their center. As you know, there is often peripheral reaction at the junction of normal and abnormal bone which *is* osteoblastic. For this reason, osteolytic lesions may be manifest on bone scans as areas of increased radioactivity!

Many radiopharmaceuticals have been employed for bone scanning in a search for the one with the most ideal physical and biological properties. Strontium-85, which exchanges with calcium, has in the past been the most commonly used radiopharmaceutical, although strontium-87m, barium-135 and -137m, fluorine-18 and technetium-99m (polyphosphate, diphosphonate or pyrophosphate) have certain desirable properties that may be effectively utilized. Fluorine-18, which is a cyclotron-produced radiopharmaceutical and at present of limited availability, has a physical half-life of only several hours and, thus, may be injected in multi-millicurie amounts, as can the ^{99m}Tc-labeled compounds. These agents allow a very high bone accumulation of radioactivity. The osseous structures will then be delineated more clearly than by microcurie injections utilized with the longer lived radiopharmaceuticals.

In the normal bone scan the radioactivity is evenly distributed throughout the osseous structures (Figure 147). Some increase may be present in the epiphyseal areas in patients whose epiphyses, for any reason, have not

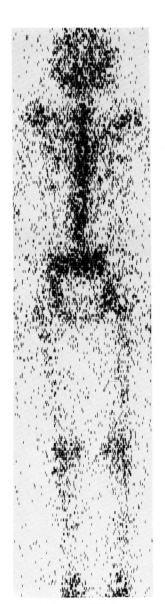

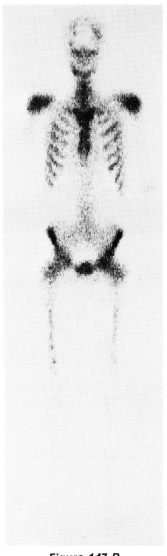

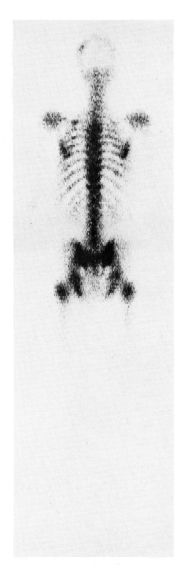

Figure 147 B.

Figure 147 C.

Figure 147 A.

Figure 147 A. *Normal bone scan (^{87m}Sr).*

Figure 147 B. *Normal polyphosphate bone scan, anterior view.*

Figure 147 C. *Normal polyphosphate bone scan, posterior view.*

fused (Figure 148, anterior and posterior ^{85}Sr). At joint articulations a slight increase in radioactivity is often present. ^{18}F and ^{87m}Sr have high photon yields, and the osseous structures are well seen. ^{87m}Sr has a high soft tissue background (Figure 149). Both are rapidly excreted in the urine. Therefore, radioactivity may be present in the renal areas and the urinary bladder several hours after radiopharmaceutical injec-

tion (Figure 149). To avoid this circumstance the patient should empty his bladder immediately before the scan is made. Strontium-85 is excreted into the bowel and may be visualized in the colon. Thus, a cleansing enema should be obtained prior to the scan.

At present the best agents for imaging the skeleton are those labeled with ^{99m}Tc. Some are readily prepared from a kit by the addition of ^{99m}Tc per-

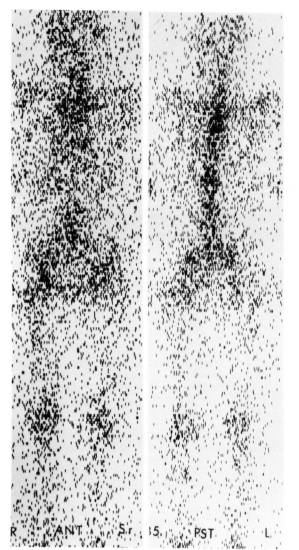

Figure 148. Normal ^{85}Sr bone scan.

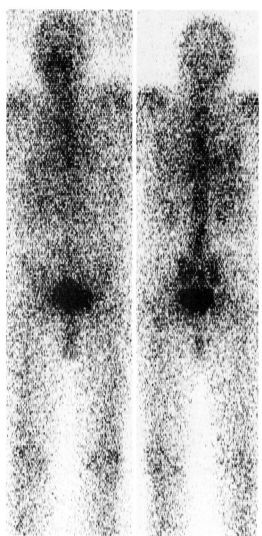

Figure 149. Normal ^{87m}Sr bone scan.

technetate to a vial. Blood clearance is slower than with ^{18}F, but good target to nontarget ratios can be achieved following intravenous injection. Up to 60 per cent is cleared via the kidneys in six hours; thus, the bladder must be evacuated to properly visualize the pelvis. Be-

cause of the favorable imaging characteristics of the ^{99m}Tc (pure gamma emission of 140 KEV energy and six hour half-life), this promises to be the most widely used radiopharmaceutical for bone scans. Better structural detail is now possible.

PROBLEM

Lena Lippman is a 65 year old woman with recent pain in the lower thoracic and upper lumbar region. This bone scan was obtained with ^{85}Sr. Are there any areas of localized increase in radioactivity (Figure 150)? Would you be aided by the findings on the spine radiographs (Figure 151 A and B)?

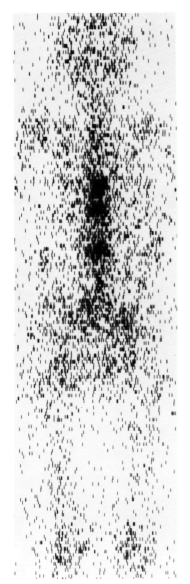

Figure 150.

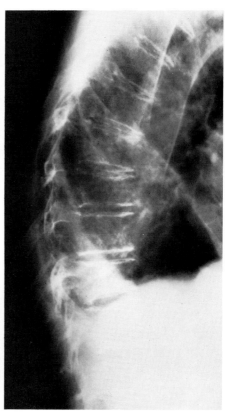

Figure 151 A.   *Figure 151 B.*

Figure 150. Mrs. Lippman's bone scan.
Figure 151 A. Mrs. Lippman, spine radiograph.
Figure 151 B. Mrs. Lippman, lateral spine radiograph.

INTERPRETATION: Several of the lower thoracic vertebrae in the scan appear to have increased accumulation of radiopharmaceutical. One can even imagine that three vertebrae are seen distinctly; this is definitely abnormal. Radiographs reveal generalized demineralization. The eleventh thoracic vertebra is diminished in its height. No actual destruction or sclerosis is seen.

In a 65 year old female what would be your differential diagnosis? She did not have a known primary malignancy.

Diagnosis: On serum electrophoresis the patient was found to have abnormal proteins characteristic of multiple myeloma. She has a pathological fracture at the 11th thoracic vertebra but no fracture in the upper lumbar vertebrae.

TEACHING POINT: Because multiple myeloma is a lytic lesion, it is generally thought that bone scans should be negative. However, our experience has been that myeloma involving bone is associated with a positive bone scan.

PROBLEM

Violet Macey, 46, had a left radical mastectomy for a breast carcinoma three years prior to her present admission. She complains of shortness of breath, lethargy and back pain. A bone scan (Figure 152) and appropriate radiographs (Figures 153 and 154) were obtained. Can you explain all her symptoms?

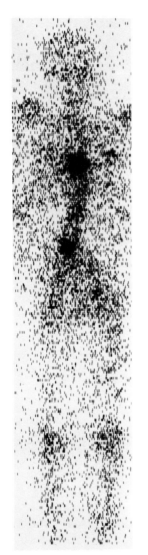

Figure 152. Mrs. Macey's bone scan.

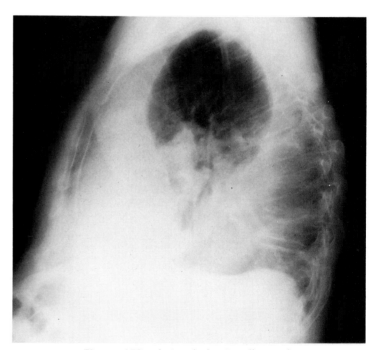

Figure 153. Lateral chest radiograph.

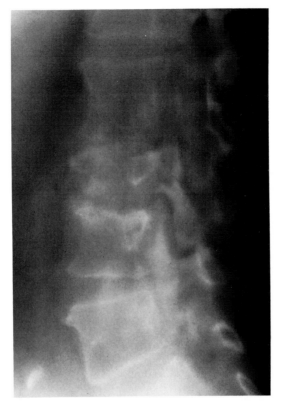

Figure 154. *Lateral tomogram of lumbar spine.*

INTERPRETATION: The bone scan obtained with ⁸⁵Sr shows areas of increased radiopharmaceutical in the thoracic and lumbar spine. There is also a very suspicious localized accumulation of radioactivity in the left chest. On the lateral chest radiograph a large pleural effusion is seen, as well as collapse of two lower thoracic vertebrae. The lateral tomogram of the lumbar spine (Figure 154) demonstrates destruction of L_3 and probable involvement of L_4, with irregularity of the bony cortex and sclerosis. Later, a rib metastasis to the anterior eighth rib on the left was seen radiographically.

Diagnosis: Metastases from breast carcinoma.

PROBLEM

John Pageant, 64, has known carcinoma of the prostate and complains of pain in his right hip. His acid phosphatase is normal. Because of his symptoms a bone scan (Figure 155 *A* and *B*) and pelvic radiograph (Figure 156) were obtained to determine whether or not *Mr. Pageant* had metastatic disease from his prostate carcinoma. Both ^{18}F and ^{87m}Sr were employed as radiopharmaceuticals. How would you correlate the radiographic findings?

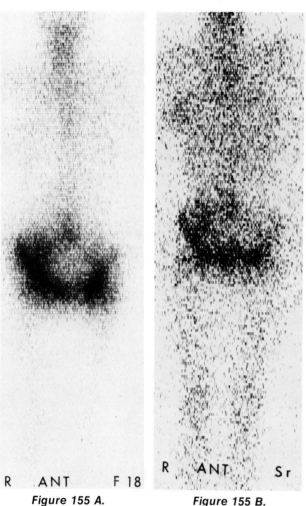

Figure 155 A.   **Figure 155 B.**

Figure 155 A. *John Pageant's bone scan (^{18}F).*
Figure 155 B. *John Pageant's bone scan (^{87m}Sr).*

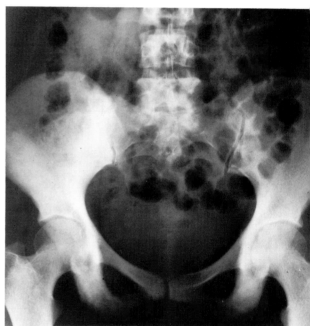

Figure 156. *Pelvic radiograph.*

INTERPRETATION: The iliac area shows marked bilateral increase in radioactivity with both radiopharmaceuticals. On the pelvic radiograph there is increased density and thickening of the trabecular pattern. However, the *iliopectineal line appears widened.* Thus, the scan is not specific, but the radiographic appearance of thickened bone is characteristic of Paget's disease. Because of the bone pain, an iliac biopsy was obtained and revealed a disorganized trabecular pattern consistent with Paget's disease.

TEACHING POINT: Positive bone scans are seen with benign and malignant disease; an increased blood supply and metabolic turnover may occur in both circumstances. Therefore, radiographic studies made of the area of interest may sometimes aid in this differentiation.

Page 130

PROBLEM

Amy Hamilton, 63, had a left radical mastectomy two years ago. She now complains of "pain in the back." This bone scan was obtained with ^{85}Sr (Figure 157). Is the distribution of radioactivity uniform? Well, in general it is, but she certainly has a very suggestive history. *Miss Hamilton's* lateral lumbar spine (Figure 158 *A*) and pelvic radiograph (Figure 158 *B*) may be of great assistance to you.

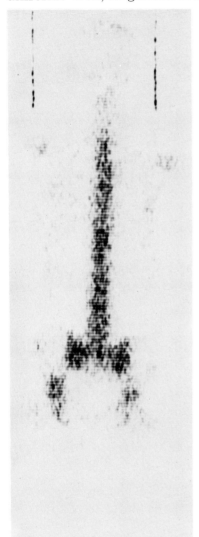

Figure 157. *Miss Hamilton, bone scan.*

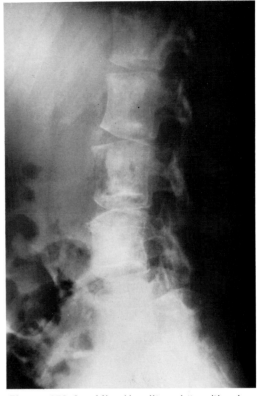

Figure 158 A. *Miss Hamilton, lateral lumbar spine.*

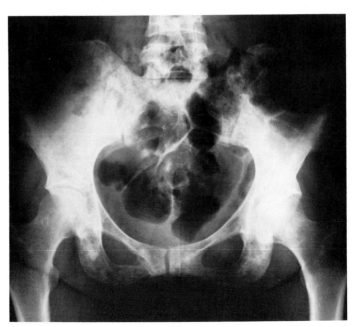

Figure 158 B. *Miss Hamilton, pelvis.*

INTERPRETATION: There are lytic and sclerotic areas *throughout* the osseous structures on the radiographs. Diffuse metastatic disease is present and the uptake of radioactivity, while *uniform,* is *abnormal.* Thus, the correct diagnosis is diffuse metastases from a breast carcinoma.

TEACHING POINT: Diffuse bone disease may show a generalized increase in radioactivity that can be interpreted as normal since very little normal bone is present for comparison.

NORMAL BONE MARROW (RES) SCAN

Since the location of the radioactively labeled colloidal particles after intravenous injection mimics the distribution of the precursors of red blood cells, these areas will be seen to contain radioactivity and reflect the active bone marrow space. Intravenously injected radioactively labeled colloid particles

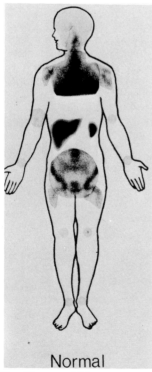

Normal

Figure 159. Normal RES scan. (From Dibos, P. E., Judish, J. M., Spaulding, M. B., Wagner, H. N., and McIntyre, P. A.: Johns Hopkins Medical Journal, 130:68–82, 1972.)

distribute not only to liver and spleen but also to the reticuloendothelial cells of the bone marrow space. Although only about 5 per cent of the injected colloid goes to the marrow, this activity can be imaged except where the liver and spleen overlap. Usually the distribution of RE cells and RBC precursors in the bone marrow is similar, but exceptions do occur (e.g., Guglielmo's disease). The spleen and liver, because they contain reticuloendothelial cells which engulf the colloidal particles, will accumulate radioactivity and be imaged much the same as on liver and spleen scans.

In the normal adult, radioactivity is present within the entire central skeleton and extends peripherally in the extremities approximately one third of the way down the humeri and femura (Figure 159). Only a small amount of radioactivity will be present in the distal two thirds of the extremities and very little in the areas of the joints and articulations. In the central skeleton, the areas of the sacroiliac joints (sacral wings) and sternum will show slightly increased radionuclide accumulation. Skull radioactivity is extremely variable. In infants and growing children some radioactivity is seen within the distal portion of the extremities and in the areas of the growing epiphyses.

Bone marrow spaces are separated anatomically by areas that do not contain bone marrow. Thus, the general distribution of radioactivity on a scan that encompasses all the osseous structures will be divided and not homogeneous, but will conform to what you would anticipate from your knowledge of osseous anatomy. However, focal lesions of decreased radioactivity within the osseous structures that are known to contain bone marrow should not be present. A focal lesion may result from any localized abnormality within the bone marrow space, such as a primary bone lesion that encroaches upon the bone marrow, a metastasis or localized trauma (Figure 160, normal and focal lesion of right pubic ramus and left iliac area).

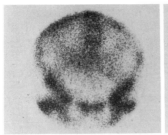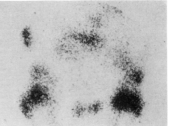

Figure 160. *Normal pelvis, and pelvis with focal lesions.*

As you might imagine, anything that decreases RES function in a central area will present as a discrete lesion. The abnormalities that are seen on bone marrow scans can be divided into categories, considering the central areas of bone marrow activity to be separate from the peripheral areas. Therefore, we can classify our abnormalities as central hyper, hypo, or normal activity and then decide whether this is with or without peripheral expansion. A generalized abnormality causing diminished bone marrow activity centrally may or may not stimulate increased bone marrow activity peripherally (Figure 161). If it does, the increased peripheral activity will be manifest as increased radioactivity within the peripheral skeleton. Generalized hyperactivity with expansion is seen on the RES scan as increased radioactivity throughout the bone marrow with a relative increase in peripheral bone marrow radionuclide accumulation (Figure 162); that is, the radioactivity will be seen to extend down the humeri and femura, and these osseous structures will be well delineated.

Interpretation of bone marrow or reticuloendothelial scans is sometimes difficult because of the limited experience with normal variations. What to expect in many generalized disease processes is not known because they have not been studied in various stages of activity. In many diseases, determining whether or not there is a response in the bone marrow may prove very useful in decisions regarding therapy and in predicting patient response and prognosis. The utility of this study will probably greatly increase in the future.

Figure 161. *Central hypoactivity (without peripheral expansion).*

Figure 162. *Generalized hyperactivity (peripheral expansion).*

(Figures 160, 161, & 162 from Dibos, P. E., Judish, J. M., Spaulding, M. B., Wagner, H. N., and McIntyre, P. A.: Johns Hopkins Medical Journal, 130:68–82, 1972.)

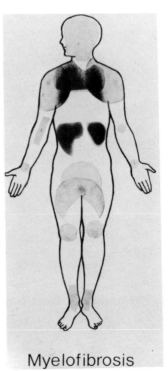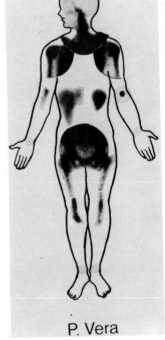

Myelofibrosis

P. Vera

Figure 161.

Figure 162.

(Courtesy of Dr. Patricia A. McIntyre.)

PROBLEM

Frances Ringer, who is known to have a carcinoma of the pancreas, is jaundiced and somewhat anemic, with an hematocrit of 34 per cent. This bone marrow scan was obtained (Figure 163). First examine the central areas. Is the liver normal in size? Does radioactivity extend below the upper one third of the extremities?

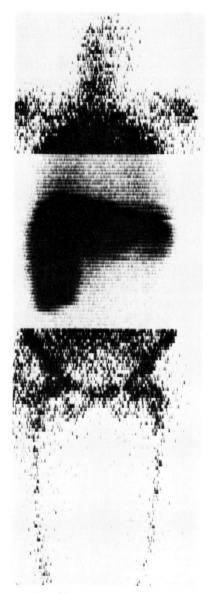

Figure 163. *Miss Ringer, bone marrow scan.*

INTERPRETATION: There is hepatomegaly with hyperplasia of the central bone marrow. Peripheral expansion is present as the RES system is visualized within the long bones of the distal lower extremity.

Diagnosis: Further diagnostic evaluation (including biopsies) indicated carcinoma of the pancreas with hyperplasia of the bone marrow and peripheral expansion.

PROBLEM

Helen Hughes, 58, has known lymphoma of the lymphocytic depletion type. A bone marrow (RES) scan is obtained to determine if there is central hypoplasia and if peripheral response of the bone marrow is present. She is anemic. From the complete series special views of the right shoulder and upper arm (Figure 164 A) as well as the pelvis (Figure 164 B) are shown. Can you answer the clinical questions?

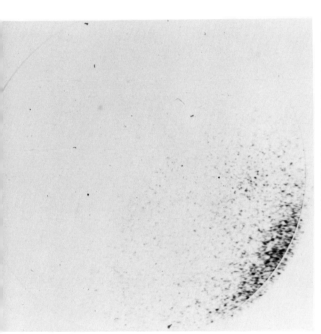

Figure 164 A. *Helen Hughes, right shoulder and upper arm. Radioactivity to the right is probably in the right lung or ribs.*

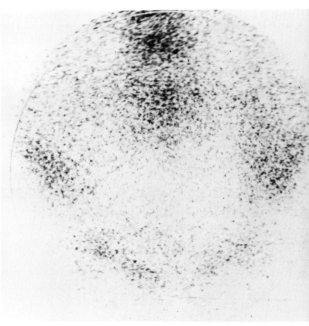

Figure 164 B. *Helen Hughes, pelvis.*

INTERPRETATION: There is diminished radioactivity in the central skeleton. This suggests that *Mrs. Hughes* has possible replacement of the functioning bone marrow with her lymphoma or an abscopal effect. Thus, she does not have a peripheral response to her anemia.

PROBLEM

Lamont Kranston, 49, is evaluated for a mass in his left kidney and an elevated hematocrit. His liver and spleen are of normal size. Figure 165 is the right pelvis and femur from his RES scan. What would be your interpretation and diagnosis?

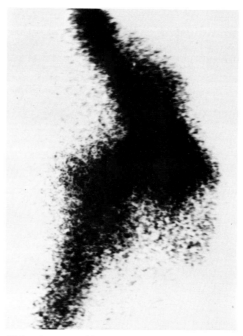

Figure 165. Lamont Kranston, right pelvis and femur.

INTERPRETATION: There is generalized hyperplasia of the bone marrow with peripheral expansion – thus, polycythemia. The mass in the kidney was not a "red herring" but a renal cell carcinoma. Secondary polycythemia in renal cell carcinoma is an uncommon but known entity.

PROBLEM

Larry Hoppmann, 66, a retired business executive, noted that he had lost 20 pounds during the past three months, felt very tired and had pain in his lower pelvis and left hip. He had a microcytic normochromic anemia and a mass in his stomach on an upper gastrointestinal series. His pelvic radiograph was felt to be normal (Figure 166). Do you agree? This bone marrow (RES) scan (Figure 167 A and B) was obtained to determine if he has had any response to his anemia and if focal lesions are present. The intensity on the camera was excessively high, giving a very dark image. Was this an unfortunate circumstance?

INTERPRETATION: The very dense spherical area of radioactivity in the suprapubic region is ^{99m}Tc in the bladder. (Some pertechnetate was "free" of the sulfur colloid.) There are focal lesions in the right inferior pubic ramus and the proximal left femur. This later was shown to be metastatic adenocarcinoma. Peripheral expansion is also present.

TEACHING POINT: Focal lesions of bone may be reflected as diminished areas of radioactivity on the RES scan before abnormalities can be detected on osseous radiographs.

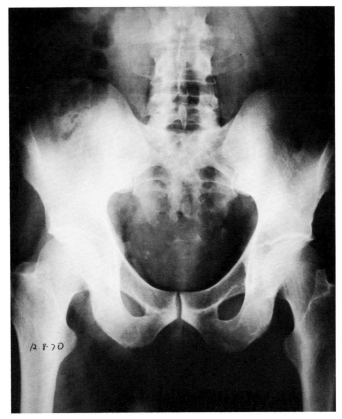

Figure 166. A normal pelvis and hip in a 66 year old white male.

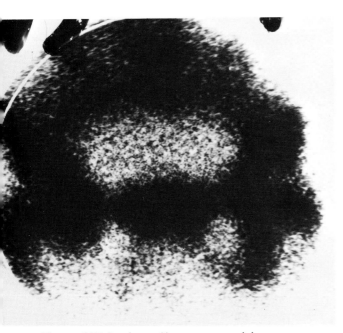

Figure 167 A. Larry Hoppmann, pelvis.

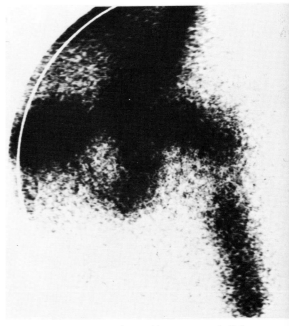

Figure 167 B. Larry Hoppmann, left femur.

CHAPTER VI

PLACENTA, THYROID, TUMOR

PLACENTAL STUDIES

To image the placenta, a label which remains confined to the intravascular compartment is utilized. Thus, the principle is the same as that of cardiac scans for pericardial effusion. After intravenous injection of the proper radiopharmaceutical (^{131}I or ^{99m}Tc serum albumin or ^{113}In) images are made over the

lower abdomen. The liver, the placenta and the walls of the uterus will be seen. Normally the placenta will be located superiorly or in the mid-portion of the uterus. If it is inferiorly located it may be over the area of the internal cervical os and represent a marginally implanted placenta or a placenta previa.

In this normal study (Figure 168 *A*) the placenta is located in the mid-portion

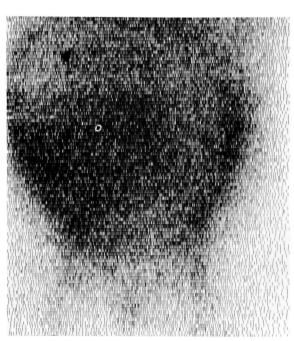

Figure 168 A.   Normal placenta.

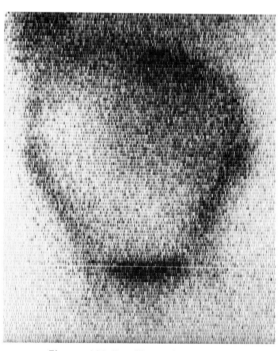

Figure 168 B.   Normal placenta.

of the uterus on the right side below the liver. The uterine walls are well visualized. Compare Figure 168 *A* with 168 *B*, which is also a normal study. The liver is seen superiorly, extending from right to left and the placenta is in the superior left quadrant of the uterus. Just below the placenta on the left is an area of radioactivity which is often present and is thought to represent the uterine veins. However, there is an additional structure in the mid-line inferiorly. What do you think that represents? The radiopharmaceutical employed was ^{99m}Tc human serum albumin. Not all the ^{99m}Tc is bound to the albumin and some is excreted in the urine. Thus, the structure seen inferiorly is not a second placenta (if it were, it would be placenta previa + twins — very interesting) but is the urinary bladder.

PROBLEM

Dora Enavant, 28, has experienced intermittent third trimester bleeding. This placental scan was obtained (Figure 169). The liver is in the right upper quadrant. Is the placenta too far inferior? Could this represent a low implantation or a placenta previa?

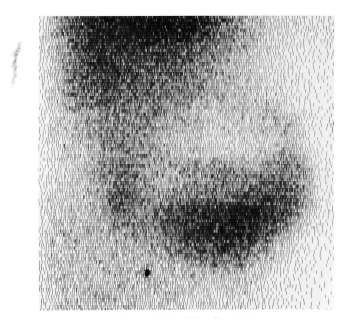

Figure 169. *Mrs. Enavant.*

INTERPRETATION: The inferior and medial position of the placenta must lie over the internal cervical os. This was believed to represent a placenta previa.

Diagnosis: Physical examination and *Mrs. Enavant's* subsequent clinical course were characteristic of a placenta previa.

Note: Although this study was very widely utilized several years ago, it has been all but supplanted by placenta localization by ultrasound.

THYROID IMAGING

Nuclear Medicine had its early impetus in evaluation of thyroid disease. The earliest images made in this new diagnostic field were of the thyroid gland because of its ability to concentrate radionuclides of iodine. The thyroid gland traps and organifies iodine. Therefore, the radionuclides of iodine such as ^{131}I, ^{125}I and ^{123}I have found great clinical utility as thyroid scanning agents. Not only can measurements of the rate of uptake and organification of iodine be obtained, but the amount of iodine within the other compartments of the body that secondarily reflect the function of the thyroid can be measured. Structural images of the thyroid gland are made following the administration of ^{131}I. Because of the high photon yield and imaging characteristics, technetium (^{99m}Tc) pertechnetate is also used for imaging of the thyroid gland. Pertechnetate is not organified in the thyroid but is accumulated within the gland in sufficient quantity to give excellent structural images (Figure 170).

INTERPRETATION OF THE THYROID SCAN

There is variability in the configuration of the thyroid gland. In general, right and left lobes, which are reasonably symmetrical in size and show homogeneous distribution of radioactivity are present (Figure 170). Since little thyroid tissue crosses the mid-line, there will be diminished radioactivity in the area between the lobes. Occasionally a mid-line or paramedian linear structure will be seen to contain radioactivity. This structure is termed the pyramidal lobe. Following surgery, irregular distribution of ^{131}I in the thyroid will be present on a scan. Some thyroid tissue usually remains.

With hyperthyroidism due to Graves' disease you will usually see an enlarged homogeneous area of radio-activity in each lobe. In some instances, because of the gland enlargement, generalized irregularity of radioactivity is present. This does not reflect nodules scattered throughout the gland or multiple hemorrhages, but irregularity as the gland increases in size somewhat nonuniformly. You will not encounter focal defects, however, if the irregular radiopharmaceutical distribution is due simply to enlargement.

In *hypothyroidism* there is a generalized decrease in the radioactivity accumulated by the gland. This is often better appreciated by a quantitative uptake determination than on observation of the scan image.

Focal defects such as nonfunctioning adenomas, cysts, neoplasms or hemorrhages present as areas of decreased radioactivity within the gland itself or at the margin of the gland. Hyperactive nodules will often be denser on the images than the normal thyroid gland because they contain more radioactivity. These nodules may even suppress normal accumulation of the radiopharmaceutical by the normal thyroid tissue. You may then image the normal thyroid tissue by administration of thyroid-stimulating hormone, which increases the function of the normal gland and "overcomes" the suppression by the autonomous nodule. Approximately 15 per cent of nonfunctioning focal "cold" areas (focal decreased radioactivity) are reported to be malignant. "Hot" nodules (areas of increased radioactivity) are almost never malignant. Occasionally a thyroid neoplasm will have normal iodine uptake and be indistinguishable on scan from the normal adjacent thyroid tissue.

Radiographs visualizing the cervical region, as well as the upper mediastinum, should be obtained concomitantly with the thyroid scan for accurate anatomical orientation. In this manner substernal thyroid masses as well as deviation of the trachea due to an enlarged thyroid may be assessed. Figure 170 B is a comparison of the images of two radiopharmaceuticals in the same three

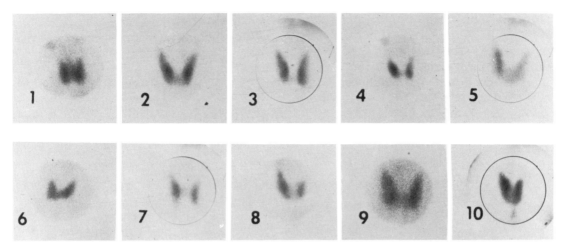

Figure 170 A. *Normal thyroid images. (From DeLand, F. H., and Wagner, H. N.:* Atlas of Nuclear Medicine, *Vol. 3, 1972.)*

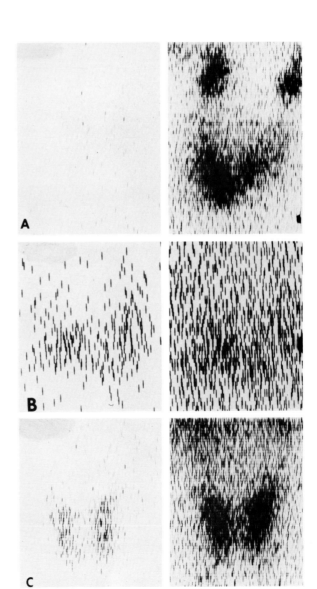

Figure 170 B. *Comparison of ^{131}I and ^{99m}Tc in three patients (A, B, and C). (From Strauss, H. W., Hurley, P. J., and Wagner, H. N.:* Radiology, *97:307, 1970.)*

patients. The first part of this figure was made with ^{131}I as the radiopharmaceutical; the second, with ^{99m}Tc pertechnetate. Because of the greater injected dose and higher photon yield, better structural detail is seen with the pertechnetate images.

PROBLEM

Judy Love, 32, is a very nervous girl who has recently noted "heart flutters." A thyroid scan was obtained (Figure 171 A and B). This appearance is certainly unusual—can you imagine any normal thyroid structure giving this image?

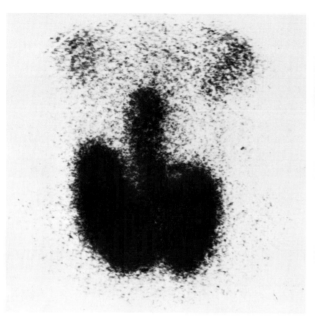

Figure 171 A. *Judy Love, thyroid scan.*

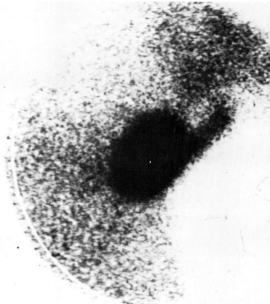

Figure 171 B. *Judy Love, right lateral thyroid scan.*

INTERPRETATION: The linear accumulation of radioactivity is in the mid-line on the anterior view and appears anteriorly located on the lateral view. As you have most likely considered, this is a pyramidal lobe. Her thyroid function tests were normal.

TEACHING POINT: The thyroid gland embryologically arises in the area of the base of the tongue and migrates downward in the mid-line to its normal position in the neck. Thyroid tissue may remain as a pyramidal lobe or aberrant thyroid tissue within a thyroglossal duct cyst.

PROBLEM

Hiram Basedow, 50, has had a 25-pound weight loss and tachycardia. Examination shows exophthalmos. The two-hour iodine uptake is 31 per cent and the 24-hour is 55 per cent (normal 24-hour up-take is 15 to 30 per cent). Physical examination reveals a firm homogeneous and enlarged gland. How would you describe the size of this gland (Figure 172)?

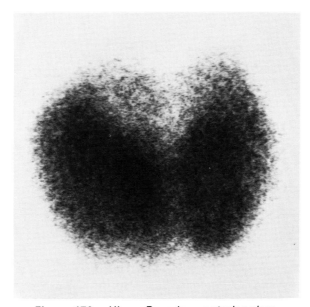

Figure 172. *Hiram Basedow, anterior view.*

INTERPRETATION: The thyroid scan shows a diffusely enlarged gland with homogeneous uptake of radioactivity.

Diagnosis: Hyperthyroidism on the basis of Graves' disease.

TEACHING POINT: A thyroid scan very clearly depicts anatomical configuration but may not accurately portray thyroid function. The apparent concentration of radioactivity in the thyroid gland can be altered by technical factors (density settings, recording speed . . .). *Thus, one should not attempt to diagnose hyper- or hypothyroidism on the appearance of the scan alone.*

PROBLEM

Murray Magnus-Levy, 38, has noticed that his hair has become dry and brittle. He suffers from constipation and feels "cold most of the time." On physical examination he has puffy eyelids and alopecia of the outer third of the eyebrows. His skin is peach colored and dry. This scan was obtained (Figure 173) as well as a thyroid uptake (9 per cent at 24 hr.; PBI, 1.2 μg/100 ml). Can you definitely identify the thyroid gland? Thyroid tissue was palpable in the neck.

INTERPRETATION: Poor visualization of the thyroid gland in a patient with hypothyroidism.

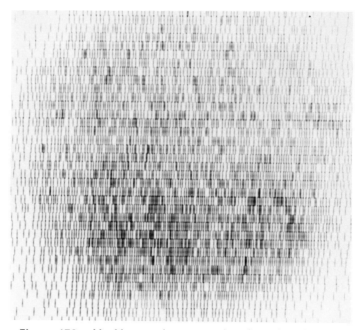

Figure 173. *Mr. Magnus-Levy, anterior view, thyroid scan.*

PROBLEM

Carole Borinsky, 17, was referred to the nuclear medicine laboratory because of a "lump in her right neck." A thyroid scan was obtained first with ^{131}I (Figure 174 A) and later with ^{99m}Tc pertech- netate (Figure 174 B). Is there a mass in the right lobe of the thyroid? Is the amount of radioactivity in that area greater or less than the remainder of the thyroid gland?

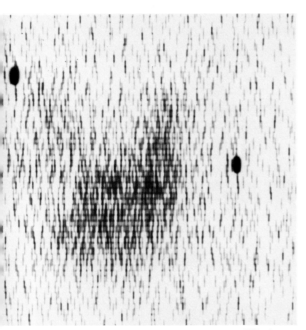

Figure 174 A. *Miss Carole Borinsky, ^{131}I thyroid scan.*

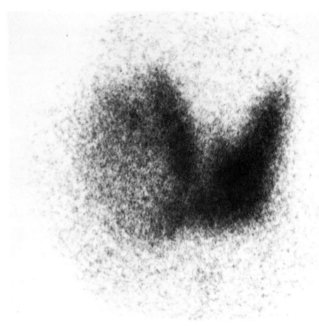

Figure 174 B. *Carole's ^{99m}Tc scan.*

INTERPRETATION: Hypofunctioning thyroid mass in the right lobe.

Diagnosis: Benign adenoma at surgery.

TEACHING POINT: Again, solitary nodules of the thyroid may be benign or malignant. It is well to remember that, while palpable nodules that show normal or increased function are very rarely malignant, approximately 10 to 30 per cent of nodules with decreased function *are* malignant.

PROBLEM

Theresa Hummer, 26, complained of dysphagia. An upper gastrointestinal series and ^{99m}Tc pertechnetate thyroid scan were obtained (Figure 175). Are abnormal structures present and, if so, where are they localized?

CLUE: The concomitant chest radiograph (Figure 176) will allow an accurate anatomical diagnosis. Is the trachea in normal position?

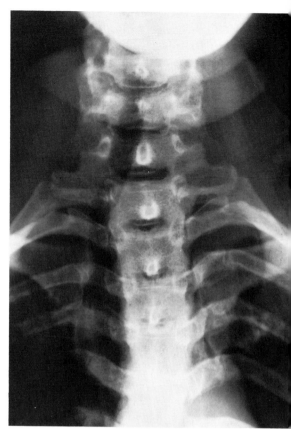

Figure 176. *Chest radiograph of Miss Hummer.*

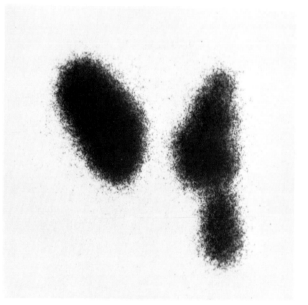

Figure 175. *Theresa Hummer, anterior thyroid scan.*

INTERPRETATION: A large extension of functioning thyroid tissue is seen projecting inferiorly from the left lobe. You detected radiographically the marked tracheal deviation which allows a diagnosis of a thyroid mass. The second scan of the entire neck (Figure 177) further orients us and places the mass in the substernal area.

Diagnosis: Substernal thyroid.

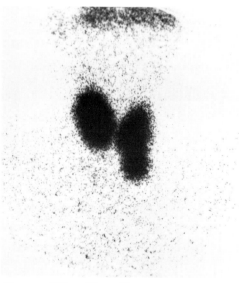

Figure 177. *Miss Hummer, anterior neck scan.*

Page 146

PROBLEM

Emily Carpenter, 34, a stenographer, had an acute febrile illness, tenderness of the thyroid gland to palpation, and dysphagia. Her serum protein bound iodine (PBI) was normal. Does this scan (Figure 178) help you to differentiate between acute thyroiditis and hemorrhage into a benign nodule?

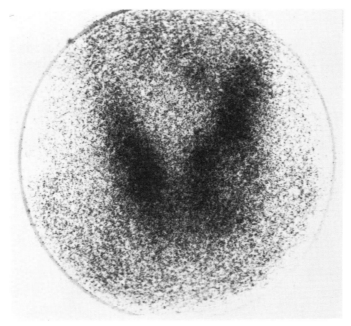

Figure 178.   *Emily Carpenter, anterior thyroid scan.*

INTERPRETATION: The distribution of ^{99m}Tc pertechnetate in the gland is homogeneous except for a single area in the left lobe laterally. In acute thyroiditis you would expect to see diminished accumulation of radioactivity throughout the gland. In localized hemorrhage (which this was) a single defect is characteristic. But *judging from the image alone,* this could still be an acute or subacute thyroiditis. The presence of the pyramidal lobe makes that diagnosis even more attractive, and one might be misled.

PROBLEM

Laura Massey, 24, noticed a bulge in her left neck that moved when she swallowed. This ^{99m}Tc thyroid image was obtained (Figure 179). Her uptake and PBI were normal. This is a very confusing study, unless you have examined *Laura* yourself. She has a firm, palpable nodule inferiorly on the left just above the clavicle. How would you then explain the appearance of the rest of the gland?

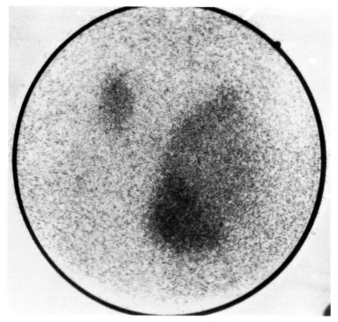

Figure 179. *Laura Massey, anterior thyroid scan.*

INTERPRETATION: This patient has a hyperfunctioning nodule inferiorly on the left which suppresses the normal adjacent thyroid gland. Stimulation with thyrotropic hormone resulted in visualization of the normal part of the gland.

TEACHING POINT: Autonomous hyperfunctioning nodules are not necessarily associated with hyperthyroidism. They may functionally suppress normal adjacent thyroid tissue. When the autonomous nodule is removed, the remainder of the gland will return to normal function, but it may take four to six weeks.

PROBLEM

Stellwag von Graefe, a 39 year old campaign worker, is referred because of weight loss (despite a good appetite) and psychic instability. (Her candidate also failed in his re-election bid). *Miss von Graefe's* abnormal physical examination included warm, moist skin of velvety texture, silky hair, eye signs of infrequent blinking and lid lag, as well as a bruit over the neck. This scan was obtained (Figure 180). Would you think that *Miss von Graefe* has the same clinical syndrome as Hiram Basedow? Are their scans similar?

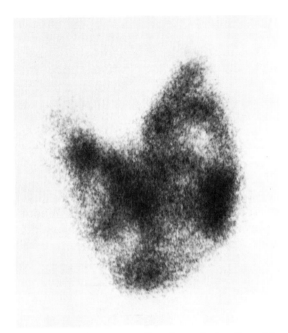

Figure 180. *Stellwag von Graefe, anterior thyroid scan.*

INTERPRETATION: The thyroid gland is enlarged and has multiple areas of diminished radioactivity. This irregular, patchy distribution of radioactivity is characteristic of that seen with a multinodular goiter. These glands usually have hyperfunctioning, hypofunctioning and cystic nodules. As these patients grow older, some of the functioning nodules degenerate, others may become autonomous and suppress the remainder of the gland while still others may undergo malignant change.

TEACHING POINT: In hyperthyroidism associated with nodular goiters the thyroid tissue shows colloidal involutional changes with hyperplastic paranodular areas that hyperfunction. Although the physiological result of this type of gland may be the same as that of a diffusely enlarged homogeneous gland, the scan appearance is quite different.

TAKE HOME MESSAGE: Thyroid imaging is a very useful procedure to determine *morphology*, not *function*. Many excellent tests employing radionuclide measurements elegantly measure specific thyroid functions. Always examine the patient yourself before interpreting the scan!

TUMORPHILIC AGENTS

Radiopharmaceuticals which specifically accumulate or are concentrated in areas of neoplasia have been sought for many years. Several radiopharmaceuticals have been employed in the past that have very high tumor to nontumor ratios. However, the emission energy of these radiopharmaceuticals was unsuitable for imaging. An example is ^{206}Bi (bismuth), which is concentrated in neoplasms but emits photons of unsuitably high energy.

It was found that selenium-75 selenomethionine will selectively accumulate in areas of increased amino acid turnover. However, the 120-day physical half-life, beta emission and rather low yield gamma photons allow only microcurie amounts of this radiopharmaceutical to be administered. Also, the tumor to normal tissue ratio is not favorable in clinical circumstances.

Two new radiopharmaceuticals have recently been employed which appear to offer future promise as specific tumor agents. Gallium-67 and indium-111 are cyclotron-produced radionuclides which may be injected either in the ionic form or as citrates. Experimental studies show that these radiopharmaceuticals probably then concentrate in the intracellular microsomes or in the wall of the cell membrane. Favorable tumor to nontumor ratios have been observed.

Although at first it was hoped that these radiopharmaceuticals would accumulate only in malignant neoplasms, reports of their concentration in benign neoplasms and chronic infection are being encountered with increasing frequency. Gallium-67 has a somewhat complicated decay scheme with three major photon emissions. The physical half-life of 67 hours allows injection of multimillicurie amounts of the radiopharmaceutical. Indium-111 has a half-life of 2.8 days and two gamma emissions of 173 and 247 KEV. Both of these radiopharmaceuticals appear to represent a progressive step in the direction of a specific tumor agent.

PROBLEM

Torrance Hugger, 54, "blacked out" while unloading a freighter at a local dock. He was found to be anemic (hypochromic microcytic). His barium enema revealed a large polypoid lesion in the proximal cecum. This ^{99m}Tc colloid liver scan was obtained (Figure 181 A). Because of the findings on the conventional scan, ^{67}Ga citrate was injected intravenously and 48 hours later this liver image was made (Figure 181 B). What are the differences in the two scans? How might they be explained by the introduction to this chapter?

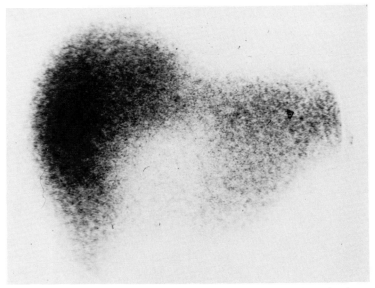

Figure 181 A. Mr. Hugger, ^{99m}Tc liver scan (anterior view).

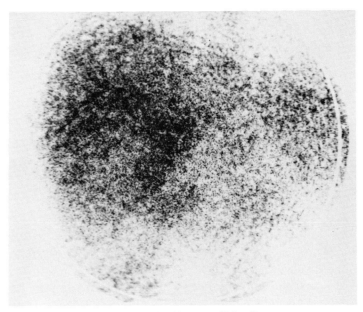

Figure 181 B. Mr. Hugger, ^{67}Ga liver scan.

INTERPRETATION: A large focal defect is present in the first liver scan inferiorly in the right lobe. The gallium scan shows "filling in" of this area with radioactivity which appears to concentrate somewhat in the previous area of diminished radioactivity.

Diagnosis: Metastases to liver from carcinoma of the right colon.

PROBLEM

Tom Swift, 26, is a graduate student who has recently completed his thesis defense. He was so tired following this ordeal that he took a windjammer cruise for six weeks. His energy did not return and he noticed certain physical signs that prompted his consulting you. From this 48-hour ^{111}In scan (Figure 182) and chest radiograph (Figure 183), can you "reason" the changes Tom noticed?

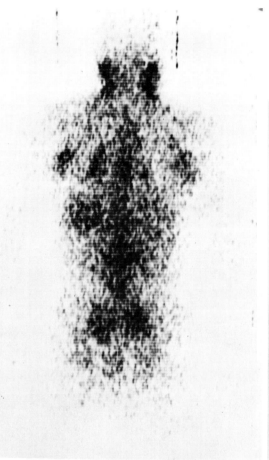

Figure 182. *Whole body, indium scan.*
(Courtesy of Dr. L. R. Bennett.)

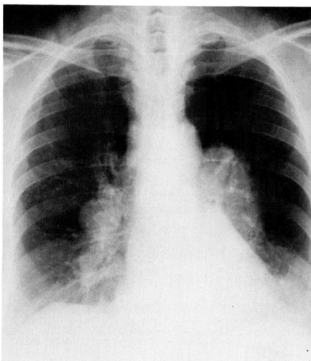

Figure 183. *Tom Swift, chest radiograph.*

INTERPRETATION: On the scan there is an abnormal accumulation of radioactivity in the neck, axillae and mediastinum bilaterally as well as in the midabdomen below the liver. The chest radiograph demonstrates mediastinal lymph node enlargement. As you have probably deduced, Tom Swift has Hodgkin's disease Stage 3B.

TEACHING POINT: Lymphomas avidly accumulate ^{67}Ga and ^{111}In. These radiopharmaceuticals may prove very useful in the staging of malignant disease, essential in proper planning of therapy.

PROBLEM

Dr. Roderick Trimble, 54, recently returned to the School of Hygiene and Public Health from an expedition sent to study blue tick fever in a lower Ubangi tribe. One of his colleagues volunteered that Dr. Trimble had used himself as a human guinea pig to test the value of gin (undiluted) to ward off the dread fever. Weight loss, right upper quadrant pain and questionable blunting of the right costophrenic angle on the chest radiograph led to this liver-lung scan (^{99m}Tc sulfur colloid for the liver and ^{99m}Tc microspheres for the lung) (Figure 184 A, anterior view). The abnormal findings provoked the ^{67}Ga liver scan (Figure 184 B, anterior view 48 hours after intravenous injection). Would you order antibiotics, call a surgeon or pray? In what order?

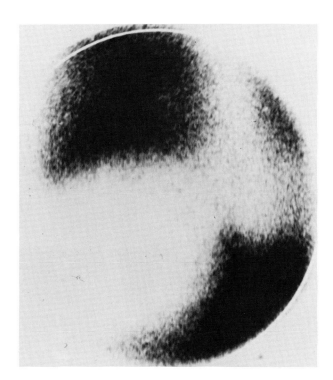

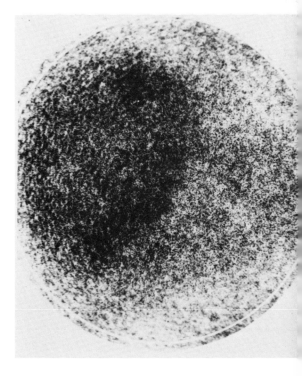

Figure 184 A. *Dr. Roderick Trimble, lung-liver scan.*

Figure 184 B. *^{67}Ga liver scan.*

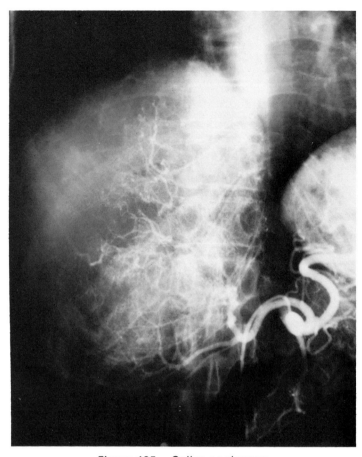

Figure 185. *Celiac angiogram.*

INTERPRETATION: The negative defect of the superior portion of the right lobe of the liver is "filled in" on the gallium scan. This is so striking that most of our clinical colleagues were convinced—that he needed an angiogram (Figure 185). The late phase of the celiac angiogram shows a relatively avascular mass with abnormal vascularity medially. A differential diagnosis of necrotic hepatoma, hematoma or chronic abscess with necrosis was offered.

Diagnosis at Surgery: Hepatoma. Score one for the gallium scan.

Comment

As we explained at the beginning of this chapter, several of these radiopharmaceuticals offer *assistance* in differentiating benign from malignant disease. If a lesion avidly collects ^{67}Ga or ^{111}In, it is probably a malignant neoplasm, although chronic inflammations such as osteomyelitis and sarcoidosis have also been reported to do so. Thus, while helpful, these agents do not represent the "magic bullet."

PROBLEM

Mildred Anderson, 86, had a Thorotrast injection approximately 20 years ago. During a routine physical a mass is noted in her abdomen. First she had a ^{99m}Tc sulfur colloid liver scan (Figure 186 A). For better characterization of the lesion an ^{111}In liver scan was obtained (Figure 186 B). Did it help?

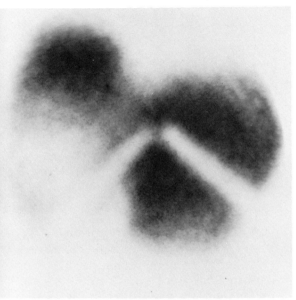

Figure 186 A. *Miss Anderson's* ^{99m}Tc *liver scan. Linear white bars are lead markers for the costal margin (anterior view).*

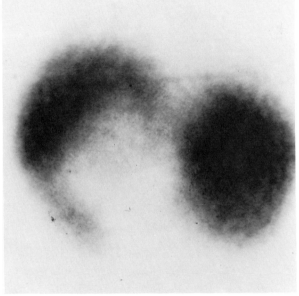

Figure 186 B. *Miss Anderson's* ^{111}In *liver scan (anterior view).*

INTERPRETATION: A large defect is seen in the inferior portion of the right lobe on the anterior view of the ^{99m}Tc scan. This does not change appreciably on the ^{111}In scan. She did not have symptoms suggesting inflammatory disease and her physicians were not prepared to believe this was benign. (Neither were we.) She had a celiac angiogram (Figure 187). Multiple densities are present throughout the abdomen from the Thorotrast injection. Minimal irregularity of the hepatic arterial branches is present, but no definite mass or neovascularity is demonstrated.

Diagnosis: At operation *Miss Anderson* had diffuse infiltration of the liver by cholangiocarcinoma. Neither the scans nor the angiograms were specific, but both were abnormal.

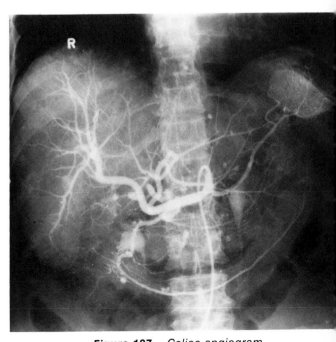

Figure 187. *Celiac angiogram.*

CHAPTER VII

BRAIN AND CEREBROSPINAL FLUID

BRAIN SCANS

The investigation of intracranial disease by radioisotopic methods is one of the most universally accepted studies in the field of Nuclear Medicine. Brain scans are employed not only as screening tests for many neurological diseases but as definitive diagnostic procedures to localize the site, characterize the shape, and document the extent of brain lesions. You will see abnormalities most commonly as increased accumulations of radionuclide in a field that contains very little radioactivity. The neural tissue itself does not normally concentrate the radiopharmaceutical and, thus, you must think of increased radioactivity in terms of abnormal increased vascularity or an alteration in the blood brain barrier. *Brain lesions cause alterations in vessel structures or in the normal physiological impermeability of the interface between vascular structures and neural tissue.*

Many gamma-emitting radiopharmaceuticals have been employed for brain scanning. However, most laboratories now prefer to use technetium-99m pertechnetate or DTPA. This radionuclide is a pure gamma emitter (140 KEV gamma emission) with a physical half-life of six hours. It can be eluted ("milked") from a technetium-molybdenum generator ("cow"). Initially upon intravenous injection, technetium pertechnetate is confined to the intravascular space. However, it rapidly equilibrates, and soft tissue, mucosal and glandular (parotid, submaxillary and submental) uptake is seen. We administer 200 mg. of potassium perchlorate orally to block accumulation of the ^{99m}Tc pertechnetate in the thyroid gland and choroid plexus. (Perchlorate [ClO_4^-] is an analog of TcO_4^- and produces competitive inhibition of uptake.) Atropine, 0.6 to 1.0 mg., is given either intravenously or intramuscularly to decrease mucosal accumulation of the radiopharmaceutical.

Many patients, in addition to having static brain images, also have *dynamic transit studies* obtained at the time of the brain scan. For this study, 10 to 15 mCi of ^{99m}Tc pertechnetate is injected intravenously as a bolus, and rapid sequence images are obtained using a gamma scintillation camera (Figure 188 *A* and *B*). This is the vertex view; it should be pointed out that many clinics use the anterior or posterior view in preference to the vertex.

The transit of radiopharmaceutical through the cerebral arteries, capillaries and veins is reflected by the sequential images obtained. Because of the rapid movement of the radioactivity, fewer photons (and thus structural information) are present on each single image. Rather than 50,000 to 300,000 counts, as may be present in the static images, only 6000 to 8000 counts make up each dynamic image. In the vertex position the areas supplied by the anterior, middle and posterior cerebral arteries are separated. You can imagine

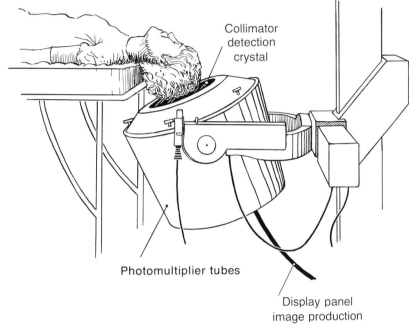

Collimator
detection
crystal

Photomultiplier tubes

Display panel
image production

Figure 188 A. Scintillation camera.

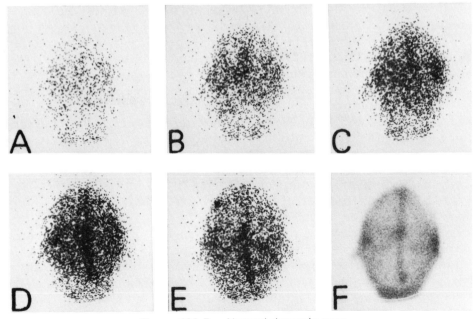

Figure 188 B. Normal dynamic scan.

(*Figure 188 A & B from Moses, D. C., James, A. E., Strauss, H. W., and Wagner, H. N.: J. Nucl. Med., 13:135, 1972.*)

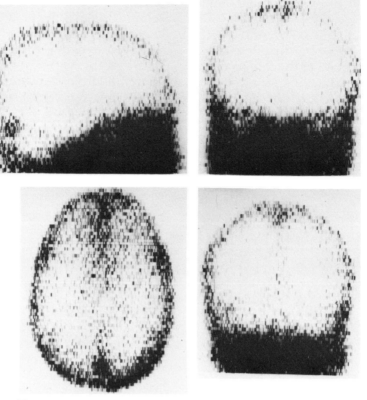

Figure 189. *Normal brain scan (only one lateral shown).*

that you are standing on top of the patient's head staring at his feet. The arterial phase (Figure 188 *B* – A, B and C) shows most of the activity in the middle cerebral artery distribution. The venous phase (Figure 188 *B* – D and E) is identified by radioactivity in the superior sagittal sinus which is seen as a linear band dividing the image.

We then wait approximately one hour and obtain the routine views for static imaging which consist of anterior, posterior, both laterals and a vertex view (Figure 189). If the static images are obtained within a short period of time following the intravenous injection of the radiopharmaceutical, the background from normal vascular structures will be greater than on delayed views. Images obtained several hours after intravenous injection of the radiopharmaceutical will have a somewhat lower background of normal radioactivity. However, these images may not demonstrate abnormal vascularity optimally.

When brain scans should be obtained is a subject of considerable controversy. A reasonable compromise seems to be within the first several hours after intravenous injection of the radiopharmaceutical if technetium-99m pertechnetate is used. We usually obtain our images at this time. The patient's head is placed under the detection crystal (Figure 190 *A* and *B*) and anterior, posterior, and lateral views are obtained.

INTERPRETATION OF THE BRAIN SCAN

On the normal brain scan in the anterior view, radioactivity in the area of the cranial vault and scalp will be clearly delineated (Figure 191). The parasagittal sinus is seen "end on" and, therefore, appears as a rather dense accumulation of radioactivity. The radioactivity at the skull base is hori-

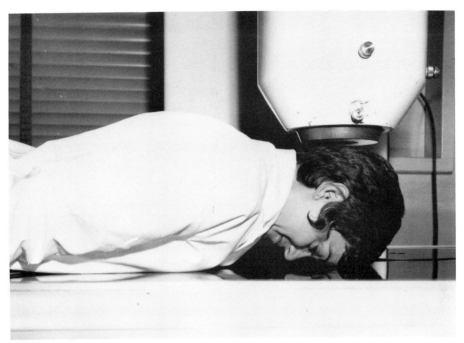

Figure 190 A. *Position for anterior and posterior views.*

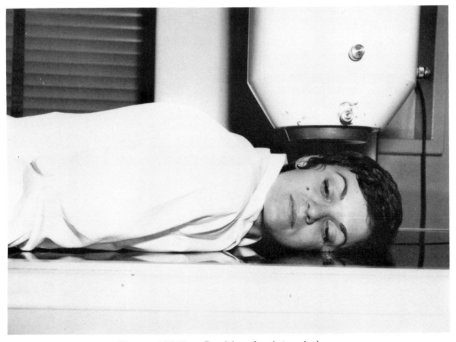

Figure 190 B. *Position for lateral views.*

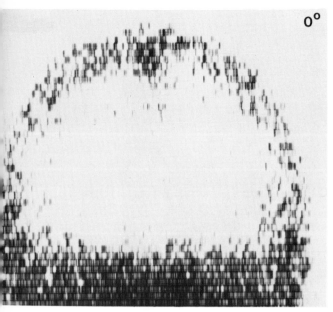

Figure 191. *Normal anterior view.*

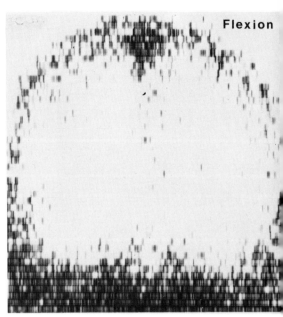

Figure 192. *Normal anterior view (flexion).*

zontal, with slight convexity in the region in the orbital roofs bilaterally. On a properly positioned anterior view or one with flexion (Figure 192) mid-line absence of radioactivity in the area of the cribriform plate is often present. Each orbital fossa is depicted as a spherical area of diminished radioactivity. Laterally at the skull base, the sphenoid wings have a somewhat upward curvature.

On the lateral view, radioactivity within the scalp, cranium and superior sagittal sinus are seen superiorly (Figure 193). This is usually manifest as a single dense linear band of radioactivity or, in some patients, as two separate lines which often correlate with a wide but normal diploic space. In the occipital region where the sinuses join to form the torcular Herophili, there is a triangular dense area of radioactivity (Figure 194). The lateral and sigmoid sinuses are curved areas of radioactivity passing from the torcular to the base of the skull in the mastoid region. The sinuses are often asymmetrical on lateral and posterior views. The right sinus most often appears larger than the left. Along the base of the skull a decrease in

radioactivity in the region of the pituitary fossa is commonly present. If all this seems terribly complex, remember the large number of structures that are contained in this small area – thus, you need to have your landmarks.

The posterior cranial fossa is often not well delineated on lateral views because of activity within the muscles of the neck. However, the region of the

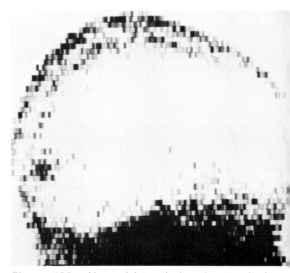

Figure 193. *Normal lateral view (anatomical variant).*

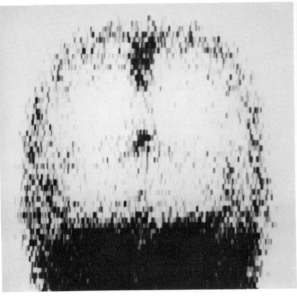

Figure 194. *Normal posterior view.*

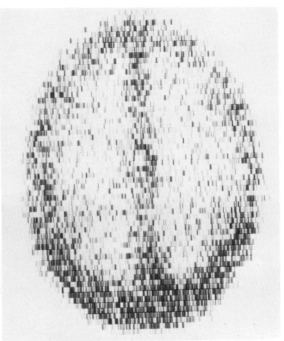

Figure 195. *Normal vertex view.*

clivus should be seen as a rather straight area of radioactivity running in a posterior oblique direction.

The vertex view is excellent for a third dimensional analysis of the position of lesions (Figure 195). The skull appears to be divided in its mid-line by radioactivity in the superior sagittal sinus. Occasionally you will note broad bands of radioactivity running laterally from the superior sagittal sinus which are most likely venous structures in the petrous area. Laterally this accumulation of radioactivity may be present in the parietal areas. Posteriorly on the vertex view some asymmetry is often noted due to the asymmetry of the straight and sigmoid sinuses. Again, this is most commonly seen as increased radioactivity on the right side.

A definite logical sequence in analyzing the various views of the brain scan should be established. For purposes of illustration in the cases to follow, the best views have been chosen and have been oriented to correspond to the manner in which we view radiographs. Therefore, the patient's left will be to the viewer's right.

CORRELATION OF BRAIN SCAN WITH RADIOGRAPHIC MANIFESTATIONS

In interpreting the abnormalities detected by the brain scan and attempting to ascribe significance to a particular lesion, you must analyze the findings on concomitant skull radiographs. Often from the abnormalities present on the skull radiograph, we can not only better localize the lesion, but can assign reasonable probabilities to the etiology. Occasionally the findings on the brain scan, when viewed in relation to the abnormalities present on skull radiographs, will allow a specific histological diagnosis.

The brain scan in the following young patient (Figure 196) is a right lateral view made with a scintillation camera approximately one hour after intravenous injection of technetium-99m pertechnetate. Because of the imaging characteristics of the scintillation camera and the vascularity of the scalp in a young child, the outline of the bony vault is well visualized. Do you think the configuration is unusual, and

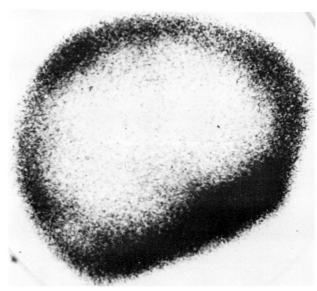

Figure 196. *Right lateral brain scan (camera view).*

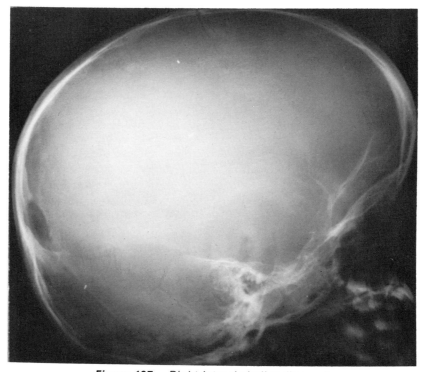

Figure 197. *Right lateral skull radiograph.*

is there prominence of the frontal area? The calvarium also appears much larger than one would expect from the size of the skull base. The skull radiograph (Figure 197) will give some indication of the patient's problem as well as the cause for the unusual appearance of the shape of the skull. What do you

think about the relation of the skull base to the vault now?

CLUE: The metallic density in the center of the skull is related to the rounded osseous defect in the occipital region.

ANSWER: The patient had hydrocephalus, which has been treated by a CSF diversionary shunt. The operative site for installation of the shunt is the osseous defect in the occipital area. The distal shunt tip, which is radiopaque, is in the lateral ventricle. Therefore, one could suspect that this is a patient with hydrocephalus which has been treated by a cerebrospinal fluid diversionary shunt. The hydrocephalus was suspected from the brain scan because the base appeared too small for the large skull vault.

TEACHING POINT: Patients often have brain scans after surgical procedures, and you must take into consideration that the abnormalities seen may be attributable to the surgery.

On the right lateral scan in this second patient (Figure 198) there is abnormal radionuclide accumulation over a large area within the parietal region. This appears to be either several lesions or a single large lesion with a cystic or necrotic center. Compare this with the right lateral skull radiograph (Figure 199).

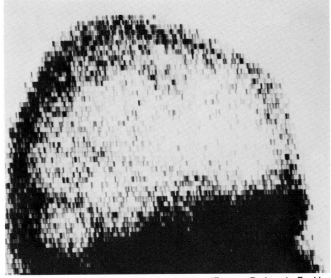

Figure 198. Right lateral brain scan. (From Deland, F. H., and Wagner, H. N.: Atlas of Nuclear Medicine, Vol. 1, 1969.)

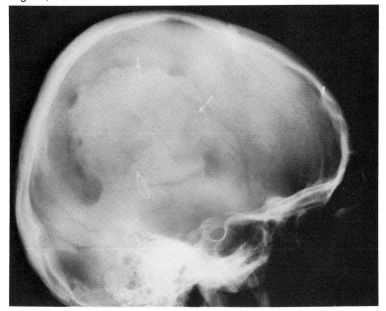

Figure 199. Right lateral skull radiograph. (From DeLand, F. H., and Wagner, H. N.: Atlas of Nuclear Medicine, Vol. 1, 1969.)

ANSWER: The lateral skull radiograph solves the mystery, as there is evidence of a rather extensive bone flap in the parietal region with multiple burr holes and sutures.

TEACHING POINT: The location of burr holes and bone flaps may be seen as increased areas of radionuclide accumulation on the brain scan for as long as several years following surgery.

After having seen the previous example, the abnormality on the left side of this third patient's posterior brain scan should present no problem in interpretation (Figure 200). Before ascribing this to the crescent-shaped abnormality which is supposedly characteristic of subdural hematoma, you should notice the left side of the posteroanterior skull radiograph (Figure 201).

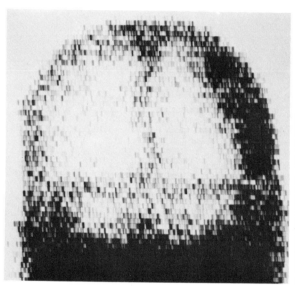

Figure 200. Posterior brain scan.

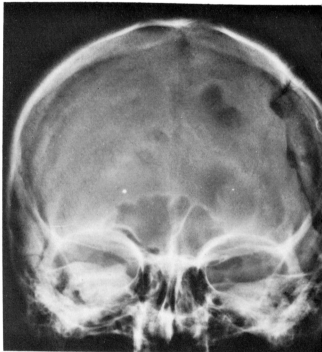

Figure 201. Skull radiograph.

(Figures 200 and 201 from DeLand, F. H., and Wagner, H. N.: Atlas of Nuclear Medicine, Vol. 1, 1969.)

ANSWER + PEARL: The cranial surgery on the left side is quite obvious in the radiograph. One note of caution is that the depth of a lesion which is ascribed to previous surgery must conform in a reasonable manner to the information regarding the surgery. Thus, if you are confronted with a deep-seated or extensive lesion in a known postoperative patient, the possibility of recurrence of the primary process or superimposed infection in the surgical site must be considered.

PROBLEM

Nathaniel A. Battle, 51 years old, enters the hospital with a chief complaint of headache, dizziness and lethargy. On neurological examination the patient had frontal lobe signs as well as an elevated temperature of 103° F. His left lateral and vertex scan are shown (Figure 202 A and B). If you would pass these as normal, we will offer a further clue.

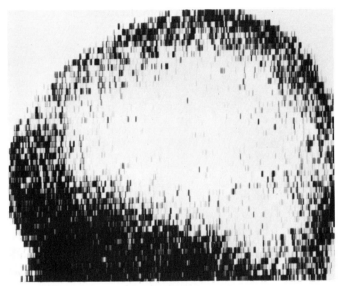

Figure 202 A. *Nathaniel A. Battle, left lateral scan.*

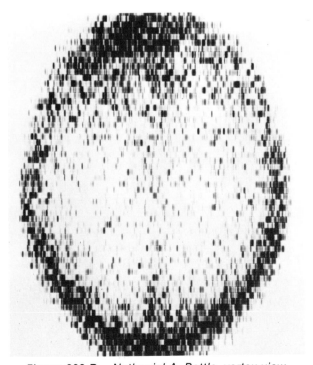

Figure 202 B. *Nathaniel A. Battle, vertex view.*

CLUE: When analyzing the left lateral and vertex views of this patient's brain scan, remember to be attentive to the peripheral areas. If this still appears normal to you or if you are not certain about the abnormality, then turn your attention to the next brain scan (Figure 203). Because of continued symptoms, this study was performed several weeks following his initial brain scan. Just as we thought, you feel much more confident about the lesion within the frontal area now. However, the major decision is to differentiate this from an osseous lesion or one within the soft tissues in the frontal area.

A selected view from the skull and sinus series (Figure 204) has been chosen because it was the only one which demonstrated the lesion. Can you delineate the margins of the frontal sinus?

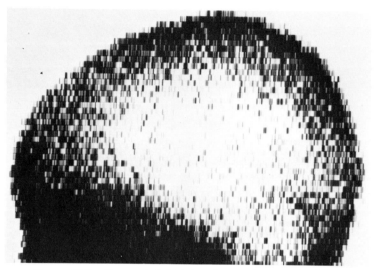

Figure 203. Second right lateral scan, two weeks later.

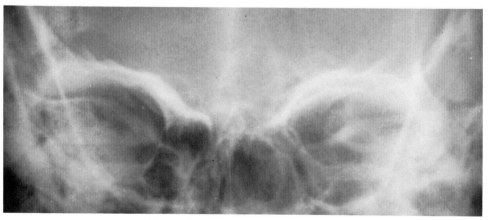

Figure 204. Mr. Battle, sinus film.

INTERPRETATION: The ethmoid sinus on the right side is normal and radiolucent, but the left ethmoid is slightly dense. However, the entire frontal sinus appears radiopaque and the margins are indistinct. This patient had a chronic frontal sinusitis which involved the posterior wall of the sinus and, then, the frontal lobe. Angiographically there was no mass lesion within the frontal lobe but inflammatory changes of the vessels. The abnormal radionuclide accumulation in the frontal area on the second brain scan probably indicates progression of inflammation to affect the frontal lobe of the brain.

PROBLEM

Related to Mr. Battle's problem is the plight of **Paul Landon,** 36, who had a frontal sinus osteofibroma removed. He developed a subsequent mucocele of the frontal sinus. *Mr. Landon* was seen at the hospital because of swelling and tenderness over his left orbit. He had been somewhat "strange" all his life; it was difficult to decide clinically whether or not he was manifesting frontal lobe signs. Correlate the left lateral scan with the skull radiograph (Figure 205 A and B).

By comparing the extent of abnormal radioactivity with the first scan of the previous case, would you feel that this anterior lesion was confined to the frontal sinus and osseous structures?

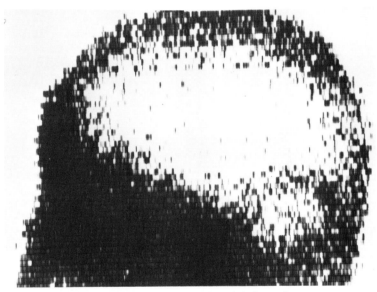

Figure 205 A. *Paul Landon, left lateral scan.*

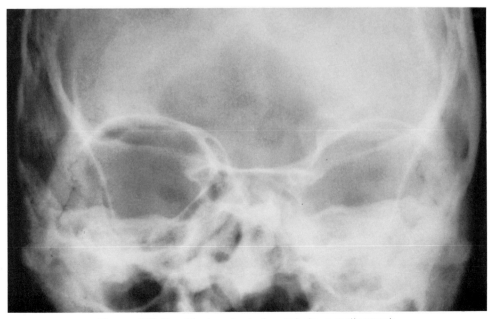

Figure 205 B. *Mr. Landon's frontal sinus radiograph.*

ANSWER: Since anatomical localizations on the brain scans are not accurate for structures less than 1 cm. in size, an angiogram must be performed. There was no evidence of inflammatory change within the vessels in the frontal lobe.

PROBLEM

Samuel Abernathy is a 65 year old man with a known carcinoma of the colon who is seen because of a puffy soft tissue lesion in his left frontal area. Does the skull lesion (Figure 206 A) compare with the scan abnormality in size (Figure 206 B)? In view of the clinical history, what is your diagnosis? Do you think this lesion is purely osseous?

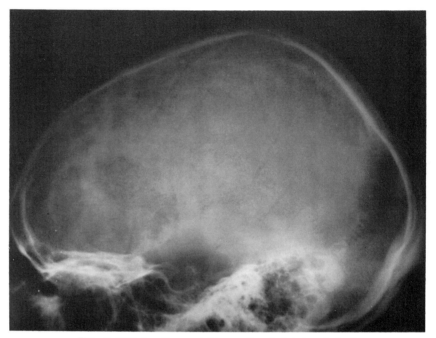

Figure 206 A. Samuel Abernathy, left lateral skull.

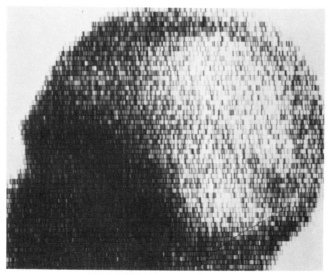

Figure 206 B. Mr. Abernathy's left lateral view. (From DeLand, F. H., and Wagner, H. N.: Atlas of Nuclear Medicine, Vol. 1, 1969.)

ANSWER: The scan lesion appears much larger than the radiographic defect. Why? . . . Should we deduce from this that the lesion is confined to the soft tissue or *do* bone radiographs and scans depict changes in mineralization with equal sensitivity? It is a widely known fact that with good quality radiographs, approximately 50 per cent of the mineral content of bone has to be altered before there are radiographic abnormalities. The radionuclide study does not require nearly so much change. This is the basis of the utility of bone scans to detect occult metastasis. Occasionally in analyzing the brain scan with the concomitant changes on the skull radiographs, one is impressed with the differences rather than the complementary nature of these two diagnostic modalities.

This lesion was confined to the calvarium and scalp. However, you could not be certain of it from this study. An angiogram or a bone scan would have been helpful to establish this as a primary osseous process.

PROBLEM

Flora Groemore returns six months after surgery for removal of a parasagittal meningioma complaining of headache and visual disturbance on the right side. In the left lateral and anterior brain scan, the abnormality within the left parasagittal region is obvious (Figure 207 A and B). This did correspond with the operative description of the surgical procedure and was attributed to the surgery. The patient was discharged from the hospital. (Would you have agreed with the disposition of this patient?)

Several months later she returns with increasing complaints of vertigo, tinnitus and diminished hearing on her left side and headaches. A repeat brain scan (Figure 208 A and B) shows again the dense radioactivity within the parasagittal region on the left. Has this abnormality increased in size since the previous scan? Because your attention is so focused on the obvious lesion is another more subtle but real abnormality present? Compare this with the first study. Were there two lesions present initially?

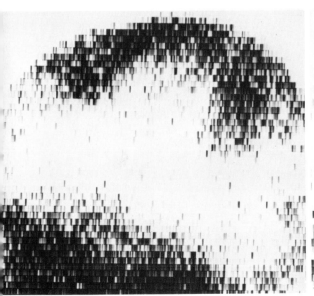

Figure 207 A. *Miss Groemore, left lateral scan.*

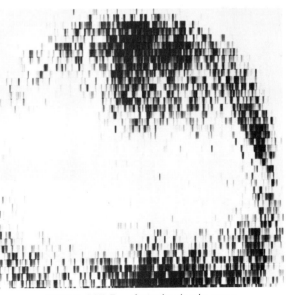

Figure 207 B. *Anterior brain scan.*

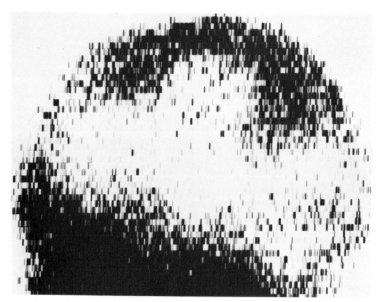

Figure 208 A. *Miss Groemore's second lateral brain scan.*

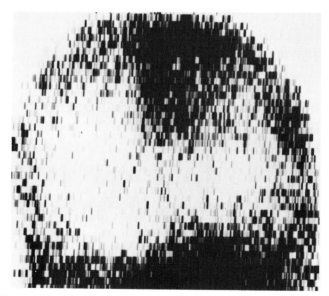

Figure 208 B. *Miss Groemore's second anterior brain scan.*

ANSWER: In reviewing the two studies you almost missed the most important lesion because you were focusing your attention on the obvious abnormality in the parasagittal region. Of course you did not miss the lesion along the base of the skull on the left side, which is perfectly obvious on the second examination and is seen, in retrospect, on the first.

The angiogram (Figure 209 *A* and *B*) confirms that there is recurrence of the meningioma of the parasagittal region, but on the lateral view (Figure 209 *B*) abnormal vessels and a tumor stain at the skull base just anterior to the siphon portion of the carotid are also present. The lower lesion was another meningioma.

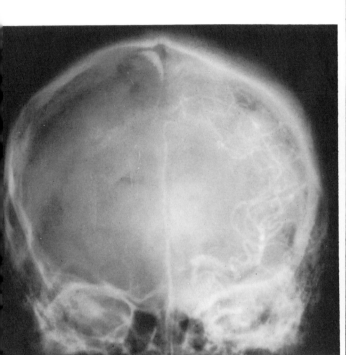

Figure 209 A. *Cerebral angiogram.*

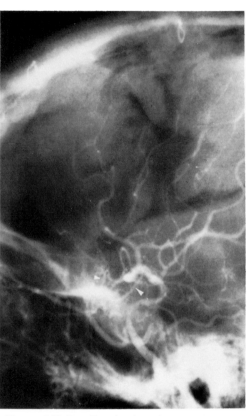

Figure 209 B. *Cerebral angiogram, lateral view.*

TEACHING POINT: First, the superior lesion was too deep to be considered merely postsurgical change, and it did appear to progress in the interval between the two studies. We should always *listen* to the patient's history; he often will tell us what areas to pay particular attention to.

PROBLEM

Miss Adeline Opporto, a 56 year old proprietor of a pizza parlor, complained of headaches, diminished vision and forgetfulness for the past several years.

This brain scan (Figure 210 A and B) and right lateral skull radiograph (Figure 211) were obtained on admission.

On the brain scan abnormal radionuclide accumulation is obvious. If you concentrate on the same area in the skull radiograph an abnormality is much easier to detect. Is the cortex of any bone particularly dense or irregular?

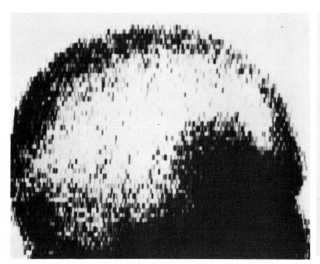

Figure 210 A. *Miss Opporto, lateral brain scan.*

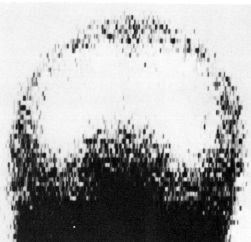

Figure 210 B. *Miss Opporto, anterior brain scan.*

(Figure 210 A & B from DeLand, F. H., and Wagner, H. N.: Atlas of Nuclear Medicine, *Vol. 1, 1969.)*

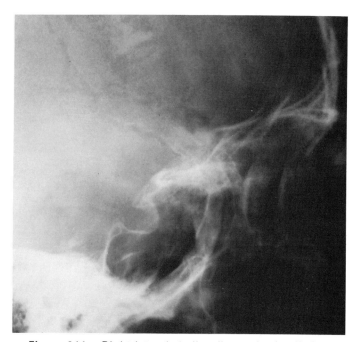

Figure 211. *Right lateral skull radiograph: detail view.*

ANSWER: Her right lateral brain scan shows a large increase in radionuclide accumulation within the frontal area inferiorly. On the anterior view this lesion is seen to lie in the mid-line between the orbits. There is intense radioactivity, suggesting that this is probably a solid mass. From the lateral view of the skull, the area anterior to the sella turcica and above the sphenoid sinus shows sclerotic reaction within the bone, with density extending upward and giving a "blistering" appearance where there should be a thin, straight line. The radiographic appearance is characteristic of that seen with meningioma within this area. This combination of radiographic and scan appearance is almost specific for meningioma.

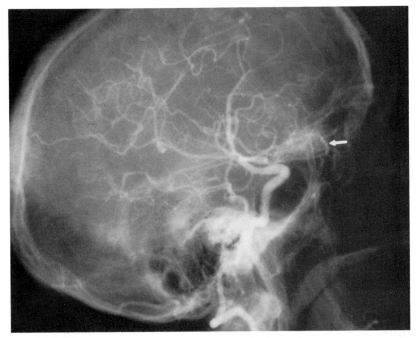

Figure 212 A. *Carotid angiogram (arrow indicates ophthalmic artery).*

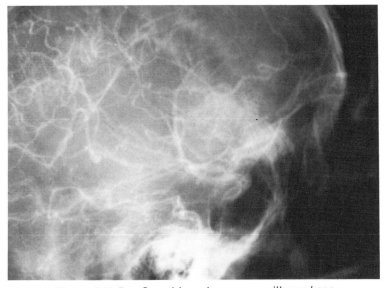

Figure 212 B. *Carotid angiogram, capillary phase.*

CONFIRMATION: The carotid angiogram (Fig. 212) shows posterior displacement of the anterior cerebral artery as well as elevation of the frontopolar branch. There is enlargement of the ophthalmic artery. It appears to contribute to the blood supply of the mass lesion which is displacing the anterior cerebral artery.

On the capillary phase of the angiogram (Figure 211 *B*) there is increased density within the area of the mass lesion owing to accumulation of the radiopaque contrast medium. This is referred to as a "tumor stain." *Hypertrophy of meningeal vessels and the presence of a persistent tumor stain are characteristic of meningioma.* As predicted from the brain scan and skull radiograph, this was a meningioma of the *planum sphenoidale.*

Occasionally the scan and radiograph are very specific. This next patient is an even better example — especially if you are aware of the patient's age and location of lesions.

PROBLEM

Rathke Jones, a 10 year old child, was evaluated because of inability to perform his schoolwork. On physical examination bilateral visual field defects were noted. This brain scan (Figure 213 *A* and *B*) and radiograph (Figure 214) were obtained. You are not too impressed with the anterior and vertex views? Well, we were only suspicious until a glance at the skull radiograph told us where to look for the subtle but real abnormality.

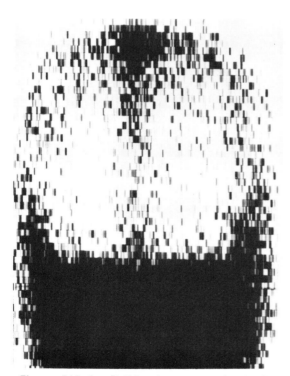

Figure 213 A. *Rathke Jones, anterior brain scan.*

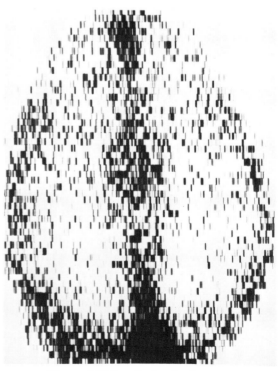

Figure 213 B. *Vertex brain scan.*

(Figures 213 A & B, 214, and 215 from James, A. E., DeLand, F. H., Hodges, F. J., Wagner, H. N., and North, W.: Am. J. Roent., 109:692, 1970.)

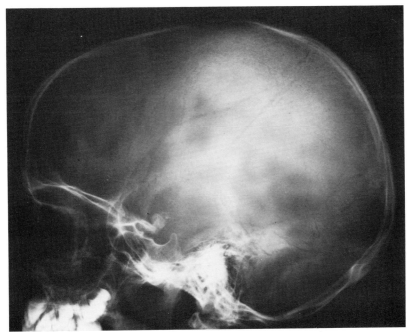

Figure 214. Rathke's left lateral skull.

INTERPRETATION: The anterior and vertex views of the brain scan have been selected because they show the abnormality. Remember that there should be a normal horizontal area of radioactivity at the skull base on the anterior view. There is a slight increase in radioactivity arising from the skull base in the mid-line in this child. We are glad that you noticed that too! A rounded lesion, superimposed upon the superior sagittal sinus is present in the vertex view. The lateral radiograph of the skull is most revealing, and proper appreciation of the abnormalities on the two studies will allow you to make a definite diagnosis in this age group with very little fear of being incorrect.

Certainly there is suggested depression of the anterior clinoid process associated with an unusually shaped sella, but the most striking and characteristic abnormality is the calcification in the suprasellar area. For these findings there are very few differential possibilities. To document the extent of the lesion, a pneumoencephalogram was performed (Figure 215). A mass is present, indenting the third ventricle and obliterating the anterior recesses. As you have correctly surmised, this is a craniopharyngioma with suprasellar extension. Craniopharyngiomas arise in the sellar or suprasellar region, most characteristically just in front of or

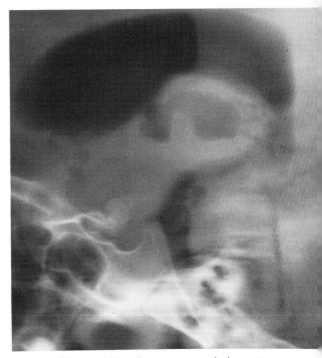

Figure 215. Pneumoencephalogram.

Page 175

superior to the sella, as they are of congenital origin from a pouch, the name of which we sometimes forget.

TEACHING POINT: Calcification in the region just anterior to and above the sella can be associated with (1) craniopharyngioma, (2) aneurysm, (3) pituitary adenoma, (4) chronic granulomatous infection, and, very rarely, (5) meningioma, (6) metastases and (7) chordoma. However, the dense character of the calcification, lack of osseous change elsewhere and the patient's age group make craniopharyngioma almost a certainty. At this age almost all symptomatic craniopharyngiomas are radiographically calcified.

PROBLEM
Reginald Lundquist, a 16 year old boy, has an abnormality noted on his lateral skull radiograph (Figure 216).The right sphenoid wing is pushed anteriorly (arrows), and the entire middle cranial fossa appears enlarged even though the radiograph is slightly rotated. This finding indicates that this is chronic process. In this age group the most likely possibility would be a cystic hygroma. A

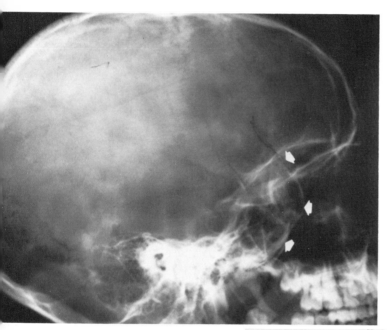

Figure 216. Reginald Lundquist, lateral skull radiograph.

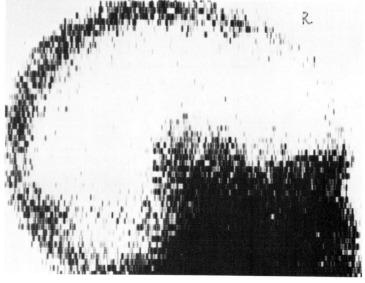

Figure 217. Reginald's right lateral brain scan.

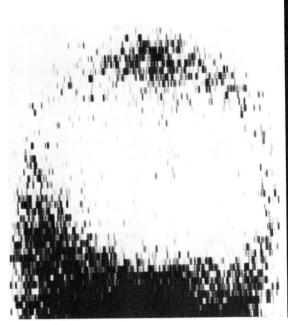

Figure 218 A. Anterior brain scan.

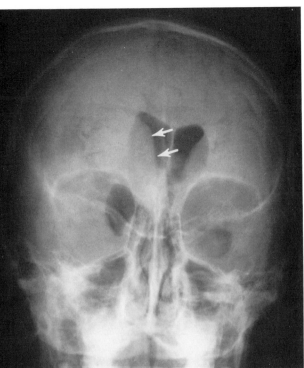

Figure 218 B. Pneumoencephalogram.

brain scan was obtained (Figure 217). With a cystic lesion at the skull base, would you expect this dense an abnormal accumulation of radioactivity? Good, that bothered us too.

Let's compare the anterior views of the brain scan, pneumoencephalogram and cerebral angiogram (Figure 218 A, B and C).

INTERPRETATION: There is a mass on the right that accumulates radiopharmaceutical on the brain scan, displaces the right lateral ventricle on the pneumoencephalogram, and elevates the right middle cerebral artery on the cerebral angiogram. This combination of radiographic and brain scan abnormalities was very disturbing; one would feel the findings most likely indicate a solid neoplasm such as an astrocytoma or meningioma. However, meningiomas are rare in this age group. Nevertheless, at operation the patient did have a sphenoid wing meningioma.

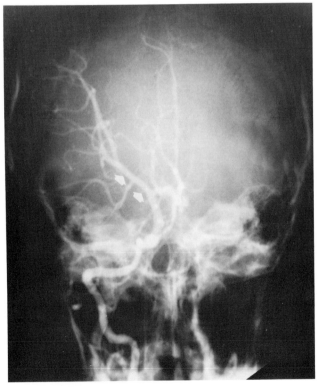

Figure 218 C. Cerebral angiogram.

PROBLEM

Bobby Dorset, 7, was admitted with right proptosis. The abnormality on the brain scan (Figure 219 *A, B* and *C*) scintillation camera is even more im-pressive when correlated with the skull radiograph (Figure 220).

CLUE: Compare the size of the orbits.

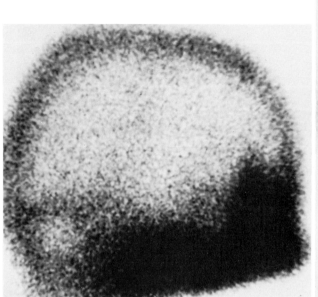

Figure 219 A. Bobby Dorset, right lateral brain scan (camera study).

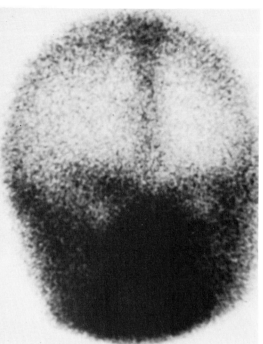

Figure 219 B. Anterior brain scan.

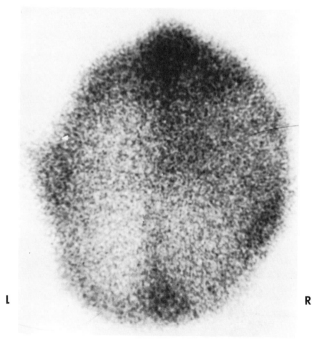

L   R

Figure 219 C. Vertex view.

(*Figure 219 A, B & C from DeLand, F. H., and Wagner, H. N.:* Atlas of Nuclear Medicine, Vol. 1, 1969.)

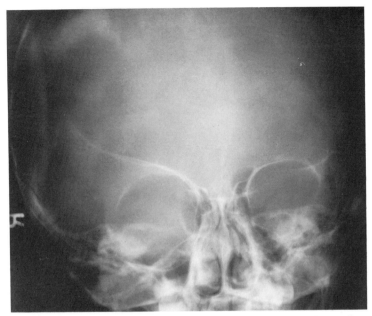

Figure 220. *Bobby Dorset, anteroposterior skull radiograph.*

INTERPRETATION: A lesion in the retro-orbital area is present on the right lateral, anterior and vertex views of the brain scan. On the right lateral view this appears to extend superiorly from the orbital roof. The skull radiograph reveals enlargement of the right orbit with elevation of the sphenoid wing and enlargement of the superior orbital fissure. Lesions such as these might be seen with fibrous dysplasia, meningioma, neurofibroma or an optic glioma.

The radiographic changes are not characteristic of fibrous dysplasia in that the structure of the bone itself does not appear to be abnormal. Meningioma would be distinctly unusual in this age group. The patient had no other stigmata of neurofibromatosis. Therefore, the most likely possibility is an optic glioma, which this was.

LOCALIZATION

One of the benefits of multiple views of brain scanning is accurate localization of the lesions detected. Often with specific localization of the lesion and knowledge of the patient's age and symptomatology, a probable histological diagnosis can be suggested with a high degree of confidence.

PROBLEM

A four year old girl, **Juanita Wingate,** was seen because of signs of increased intracranial pressure and ataxia. The left lateral and posterior views of the brain scan are shown (Figure 221 A and B, anterior and lateral). Can you localize the abnormality? In this age group, what are the possibilities?

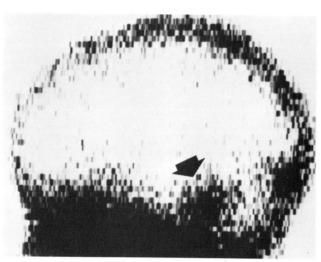

Figure 221 A.   *Left lateral view.*   **Figure 221 B.**   *Posterior view.*

(Figure 221 A & B from DeLand, F. H., and Wagner, H. N.: Atlas of Nuclear Medicine, Vol. 1, 1969.)

INTERPRETATION: This lesion appears to lie below the tentorium of the cerebellum and in the mid-line, thus localizing it to the fourth ventricle or the vermis of the cerebellum. Particularly common in this age group are medulloblastomas. A cystic astrocytoma would more often occur in the cerebellar hemispheres and is usually seen in slightly older children. Ependymoma is more uncommon and the average age of occurrence is older. Pontine gliomas are much closer to the skull base, and chordomas are usually superior in location along the clivus.

CONFIRMATION: The pneumoencephalogram and the cerebral angiogram showed signs of a lesion in the cerebellar area but did not characterize the lesion any better than the brain scan. At surgical exploration of the posterior fossa, a medulloblastoma was present.

TEACHING POINT: A mid-line lesion in the cerebellar area in this age group is most likely to be a medulloblastoma. If the patient had been a few years older or the lesion had been in the more lateral cerebellar area, cystic astrocytoma would have been an equally likely diagnostic possibility. Had the lesion blended into the radioactivity at the skull base along the area of the clivus, a pontine glioma should have been considered. The location of a chordoma is more superior, and radiographically abnormalities of the clivus or calcification in that area may be present.

PROBLEM

Victor Malone, 55, had a chief complaint of ringing in his ears and loss of hearing on the right side. He had a brain scan (Figure 222 A, B and C). After identifying the lesion can you localize it to a specific area? Because of the abnormality on the brain scan, the patient's history and the questionable abnormality on the Townes view of the skull radiograph (Figure 223), tomograms of the internal auditory canal were obtained. Do the two internal auditory canals appear symmetrical (Figure 224)? Can you outline the roof and the floor on each side?

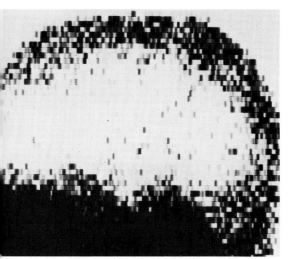

Figure 222 A. *Victor Malone, right lateral brain scan.*

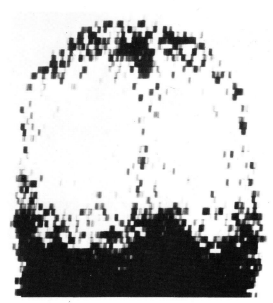

Figure 222 B. *Posterior brain scan.*

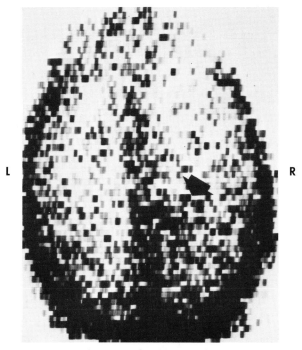

Figure 222 C. *Vertex view.*

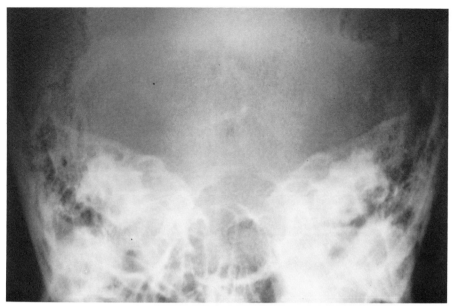

Figure 223. Townes view of skull.

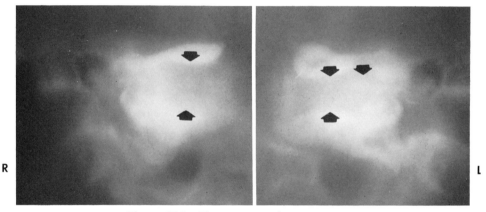

R   L

Figure 224. Tomograms of petrous areas.

INTERPRETATION: The static brain scan shows a lesion at the right cerebellopontine angle. Skull radiographs and tomograms of the internal auditory canal demonstrate widening of this structure on the right side, with loss of the bony cortex of the floor. Almost all such lesions are acoustic neurinomas, as this one was. It is, therefore, very important in interpreting the brain scan to be as specific as possible in localizing the lesion to the cerebellopontine angle.

PROBLEM

Libby Franks, a 48 year old advertising executive, has been having headaches for five years. She has been afebrile. Her skull radiographs were normal, but she had a mid-line focus on her electro-encephalogram. Both the lateral and anterior view of the brain scan are shown, as well as a series of "tomographic" views (Figure 225 A, B, C and D). Localize the lesion and consider the possibilities in a middle-aged patient.

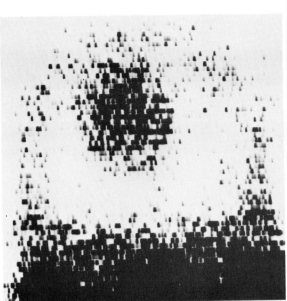

Figure 225 A. *Miss Franks, anterior view brain scan.*

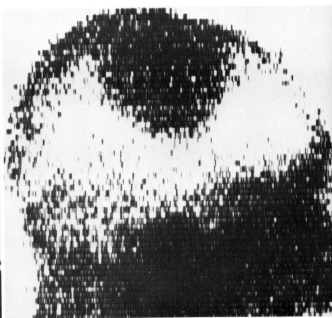

Figure 225 B. *Right lateral brain scan.*

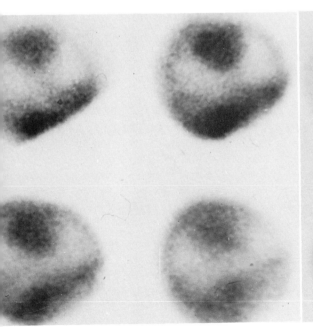

Figure 225 C. *Right lateral tomographic scan.*

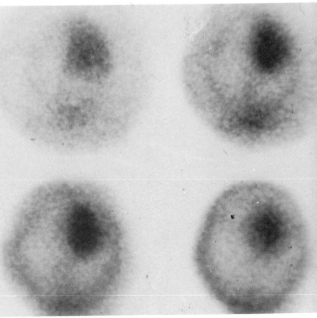

Figure 225 D. *Vertex tomogram.*

(Figure 225 A, B & C from Chamroenngan, S., Langan, J. K., Trattner, J. M., Muellehner, G., and Wagner, H. N.: Radiology, 98:445, 1971.*)*

INTERPRETATION: The anterior and lateral views of the brain scan show a large lesion just to the right of the mid-line and superior in location. A rounded lesion in this parasagittal location in a middle-aged patient, especially a female, with a longstanding clinical history is very suggestive of one particular diagnosis.

Occasionally the location of lesions is greatly assisted by special views or techniques. Tomographic scans may be obtained in much the same way as tomographic radiographs. The plane of optimum resolution, or "focus," is thus selected. The tomograms in multiple views allow depth localization. By computing the plane of best resolution in two views, the true location of the lesion can be determined.

This is a lesion adjacent to the midline that is spherical in shape and is, most likely then, a neoplasm or abscess. The patient had a long history but no temperature elevation. Considering the location and clinical circumstance, it should then be . . .

Diagnosis: Falx meningioma, which is well demonstrated on the cerebral angiogram (Figure 226). Displacement of the anterior cerebral artery and abnormal vessels with a tumor blush or stain is present.

PEARL: Location along the falx increases the probability of meningioma, and meningiomas are more common in females.

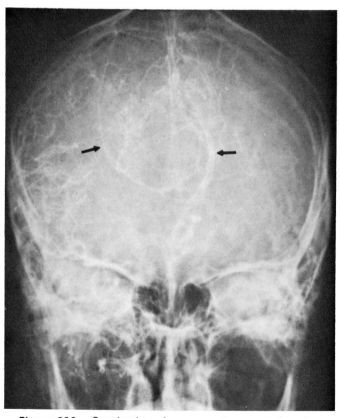

Figure 226. Cerebral angiogram, anteroposterior view.

PROBLEM

George "Bruiser" Goforth, 47, finished second in an altercation only a few yards from the emergency room entrance. However, he delayed coming to the hospital because he "felt fine" the next day. He had been struck in the occipital region and on the left side posteriorly. A brain scan (Figure 227 A and B) was performed 10 days following trauma.

(Note: The posterior here is oriented as the scanner "sees" the patient, a departure from our usual procedure but utilized in some laboratories. Where would you localize this lesion? In view of his history of trauma you would be quite interested in the findings on the skull radiograph, but no fracture was seen.)

L   R

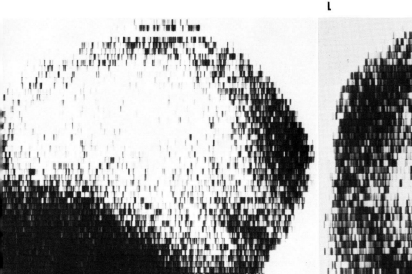 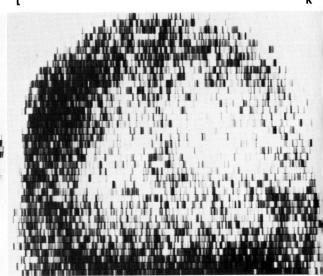

Figure 227 A. *George Goforth, left lateral brain scan.*

Figure 227 B. *Mr. Goforth, posterior view (seen from behind).*

INTERPRETATION: The left lateral and posterior views show a large abnormal concentration of the radiopharmaceutical peripherally and posteriorly. From the posterior view this has a somewhat "crescentic" configuration.

As I am certain you have deduced from the peripheral nature of the lesion and its crescentic shape, a subdural hematoma is the primary diagnosis to be considered. The clinical history is also excellent for this, but to establish the diagnosis a cerebral angiogram must be obtained. The angiogram (Figure 228, capillary phase) shows displacement of the vessels from the inner table of the calvarium characteristic of a subdural hematoma, probably chronic:

Diagnosis: Subdural hematoma.

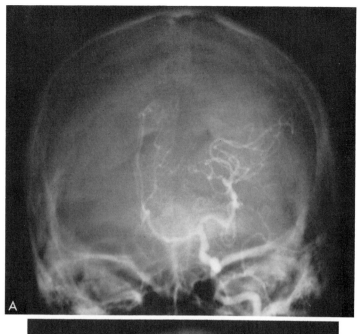

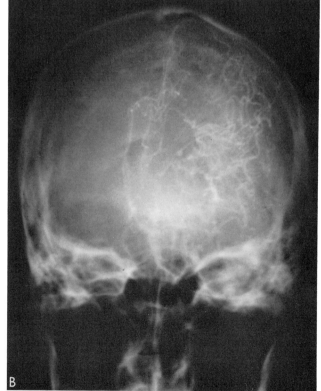

Figure 228. Cerebral angiogram.

PROBLEM

Grant Malinger, 52, was at work when he "fainted." When he regained consciousness, a matter of minutes later, *Grant* had a neurological abnormality consisting of paralysis and a sensory deficit of the right leg. In questioning his fellow employees his physician learned that he had had several episodes of forgetfulness and motor apraxia over the preceding months. The skull radiographs were normal. He had a brain scan (Figure 229 A and B) seven days after the onset of paralysis.

Does the lesion on the anterior view correspond to what you would expect from the left lateral view? If it does not, it should suggest that the lesion is diffuse or multiple or medial in location, or both. Placing the findings on the brain scan in relation to the clinical history, what would be your primary diagnosis? Now let's have a look at two views of the cerebral angiogram to see if you were correct specifically or generally.

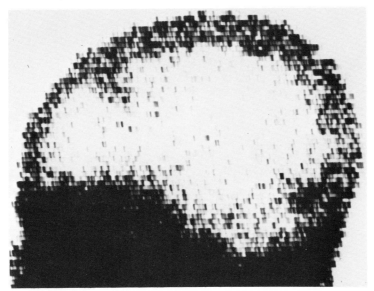

Figure 229 A. *Grant Malinger, left lateral view, brain scan.*

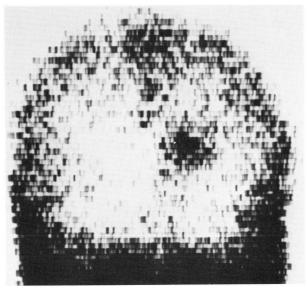

Figure 229 B. *Grant Malinger, anterior view, brain scan.*
(Figure 229 A & B from DeLand, F. H., and Wagner, H. N.: Atlas of Nuclear Medicine, *Vol. 1,* 1969.)

CEREBRAL ANGIOGRAM (Figure 230): Contrast material is seen to enter only the most proximal portion of the anterior cerebral artery (arrow). The middle cerebral circulation fills out well with contrast medium.

Diagnosis: Anterior cerebral artery occlusion with probable infarction.

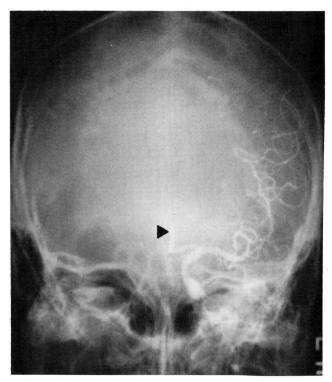

Figure 230 A. *Mr. Malinger's cerebral angiogram.*

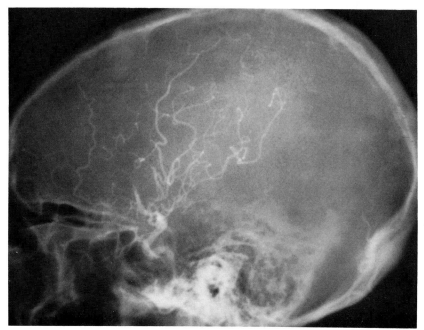

Figure 230 B. *Mr. Malinger's left lateral angiogram.*
(Figure 230 A & B from DeLand, F. H., and Wagner, H. N.: Atlas of Nuclear Medicine, Vol. 1, 1969.)

RADIOPHARMACEUTICAL ACCUMULATION AND APPEARANCE

Characterization of the manner in which the abnormality accumulates the radiopharmaceutical may be of significance. Equally important is the temporal sequence of radiopharmaceutical disappearance from the lesion. For this assessment you should obtain dynamic studies and, occasionally, delayed images.

Neoplasms can usually be differentiated from cerebral infarctions by a combination of static and dynamic brain images. *If you delineate a lesion on the static image which shows diminished radioactivity in that area on the dynamic study, it is most likely a cerebral infarction. Neoplasms will usually be seen as abnormal accumulations of radioactivity on the static study and normal or increased areas of radioactivity on the dynamic study.*

There are lesions which have increased radioactivity on the dynamic study. They may sometimes be differentiated from each other by the manner in which radiopharmaceutical accumulates and disappears.

For example, arteriovenous malformations show early increase of radionuclide accumulation with diminished radioactivity in the late venous phase of the dynamic study. On the other hand, a glioblastoma multiforme usually shows radionuclide accumulation which does not appear quite so early as in an A-V malformation, and the clearing of the radiopharmaceutical does not appear so definite on the venous phase. Meningiomas do not have as early an appearance as either of the two lesions just mentioned but show progressive increase in radioactivity throughout the venous phase. These changes in sequence as the radionuclide passes from the arterial to the venous circulation allow you to offer a probability statement regarding the various diagnostic possibilities. Before attempting the following cases, you might want to review the normal dynamic study (Figure 188 *B*).

PROBLEM

This patient, **Felix Mitchell,** a 65 year old man, had a two-month history of right arm weakness. He is now aphasic and has a right hemiplegia. These neurological deficits have been progressive.

The static brain scan and dynamic transit study in the vertex position were obtained on his admission. Would you characterize the lesion on the static image (Figure 231 *A* and *B* posterior and vertex) as diffuse or localized? Does it correspond to any normal vascular distribution? Does it have homogeneous accumulation of the radiopharmaceutical? Now that you have answered these queries, examine the radionuclide transit study (Figure 232 *A* and *B*, arterial and capillary phases). Remember that the vertex view reveals the cerebral circulation as if you were standing on top of the patient's skull peering down.

INTERPRETATION: The posterior and vertex views of the static study reveal a large spherical lesion posteriorly on the left side with a center that does not contain as much radioactivity as the periphery. On the cerebral transit study the increased radioactivity at 5 o'clock is from the injection bolus (right carotid). The left-sided lesion accumulates radioactivity in the early phase and is very well seen before the superior sagittal sinus is delineated. There was no "clearing" of the radioactivity in this abnormal area on later images of the dynamic study.

Considering the patient's age, the size of the lesion, and the characteristics of radionuclide transit through it, the differential diagnosis is quite limited. This pattern, common for astrocytoma Grade IV (glioblastoma multiforme), is uncommonly encountered with A-V malformations, and may rarely be seen in very vascular meningiomas.

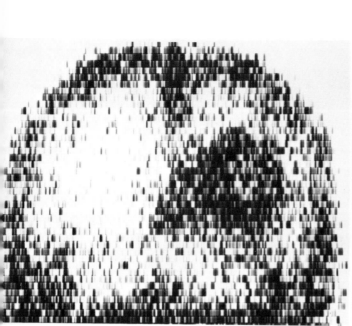

Figure 231 A. *Mr. Mitchell, posterior brain scan.*

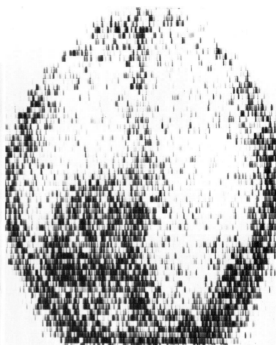

Figure 231 B. *Felix Mitchell, vertex view.*

L   R L   R

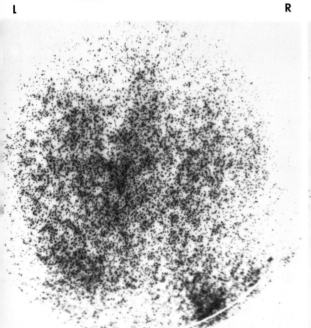

Figure 232 A. *Dynamic transit study (arterial phase).*

Figure 232 B. *Dynamic transit study (capillary phase).*

Cerebral angiography (Figure 233 *A* and *B*) shows markedly abnormal vessels in the parietal area, irregular caliber of vessels and "pooling" of contrast in neoplastic sinusoids. Early venous drainage from the area is seen (arrows). This pattern is diagnostic of glioblastoma multiforme.

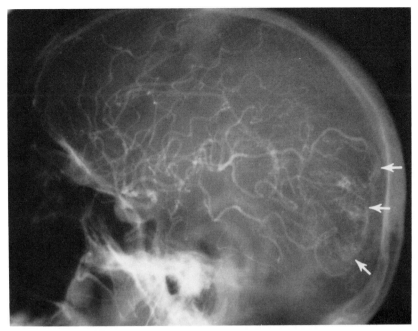

Figure 233 A. *Mr. Mitchell, cerebral angiogram (lateral view).*

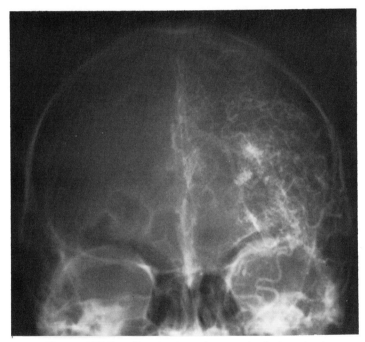

Figure 233 B. *Cerebral angiogram (anterior view).*

TEACHING POINT: If a lesion early in the dynamic study has greater radioactivity than the corresponding normal brain tissue, it suggests that it has an enlarged blood supply or is primarily vascular. When the superior sagittal sinus is seen as a linear density of radioactivity, the venous phase is predominating. If the lesion continues to become more intense after this time period it is more likely a meningioma. Consider the next patient. . . .

PROBLEM

Matilda Governeur. The vertex view of the venous phase of her radionuclide cerebral angiogram (Figure 234) is virtually diagnostic. Intense abnormal radioactivity which appears to increase during the later phases of the study in a middle-aged woman should suggest . . .

well, yes, that a cerebral angiogram should be obtained! *Matilda* had had transient periods of bizarre behavior for several years prior to the brain scan. Here, the cerebral angiogram (Figure 235 *A* and *B*) is even more specific.

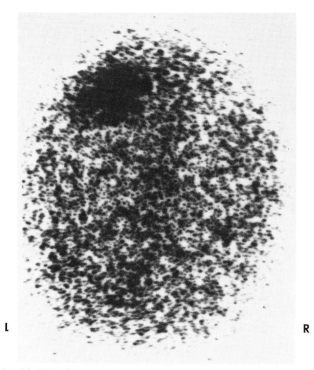

L   R

Figure 234. Matilda Governeur, vertex view (venous phase), dynamic study.

INTERPRETATION: The left lateral view of the angiogram confirms the impression of a mass anteriorly in the left frontal lobe. Abnormally large and irregular meningeal vessels (arrow) are present, supplying the lesion. The intense homogeneous contrast "stain" suggests meningioma. This homogene-ous concentration of contrast on the capillary and venous phases of the angiogram corresponds to the dense accumulation of radioactivity on the later phases of the radionuclide cerebral transit study.

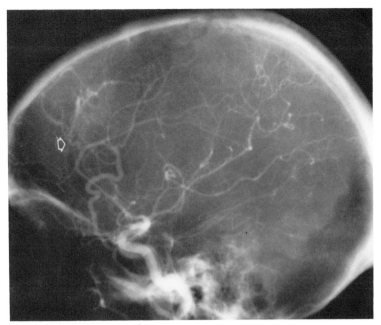

Figure 235 A. *Left lateral view, cerebral angiogram.*

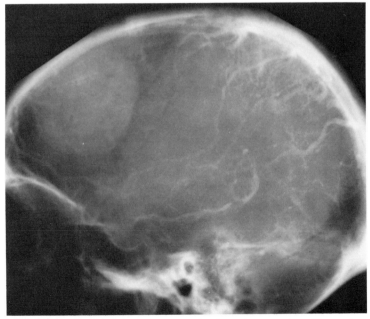

Figure 235 B. *Left lateral view, cerebral angiogram (capillary phase).*

PROBLEM

Clara Velda Arthur had a sudden "attack" resulting in a right hemiplegia. Her skull radiographs and initial static brain scan performed within hours of the onset of symptoms were normal.

Because of the clinical history a dynamic study was obtained in the vertex position (Figure 236 *A*, early, and late venous phase, *B*).

L   R   L

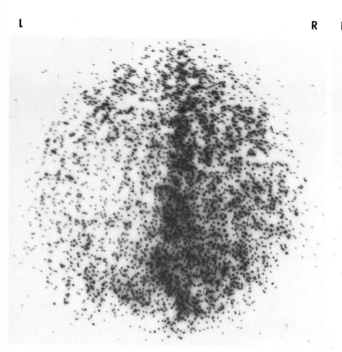 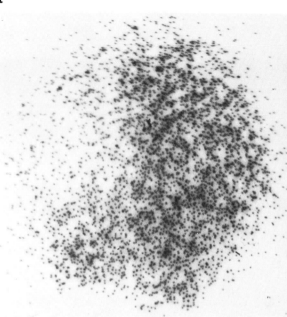

Figure 236 A. *Mrs. Arthur, dynamic study, early venous phase.*

Figure 236 B. *Mrs. Arthur, late venous phase.*

CLUE: Remember perfusion of the cerebral hemispheres should be equal. Is that true here? What are the diagnostic possibilities? Do any of these diagnoses agree with the clinical story?

INTERPRETATION: On the early venous images, decreased radioactivity to the central part of the entire left hemisphere is present. This abnormal finding persisted throughout the study. The most common cause of this appearance is a middle cerebral artery occlusion. An angiogram confirmed that a middle cerebral artery thrombosis had indeed occurred. Her static brain scan became positive approximately one week after the initial study. The temporal sequence of events is characteristic of cerebrovascular thrombosis or occlusion.

Delayed studies are used to delineate avascular lesions, especially metastases, but also to better characterize certain other types of lesions. The ability of a lesion to continue to concentrate radionuclide on delayed views taken hours after intravenous injection sometimes correlates with a tumor "stain" at angiography.

PROBLEM

Mr. Perry Carmichael, 46, had a seizure and was left with a right hemiparesis. The scan was performed three days after onset of symptoms (Figure 237).

This lesion is very active on the ini-tial left lateral scan. On the two delayed views (Figure 238 *A* and *B*) compare the activity in the buccal mucosa with that in the lesion.

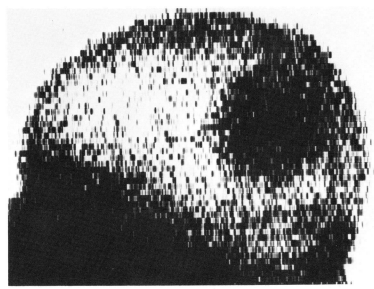

Figure 237. *Mr. Perry Carmichael, left lateral scan.*

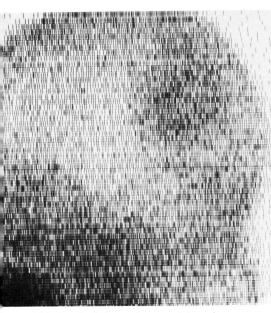

gure 238 A. *Left lateral scan at four hours.*

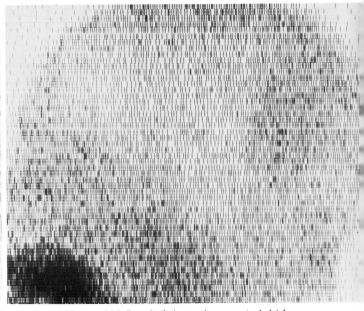

Figure 238 B. *Left lateral scan at eight hours.*

INTERPRETATION: A large parietal lè-sion is present in the left hemisphere on the initial scan. At four hours the radio-pharmaceutical accumulation in the lesion is diminishing at approximately the same rate as normal vascular struc-tures. By eight hours (Figure 238 *B*) the radioactivity in the parotid gland and buccal mucosa is much greater than in the lesion. The shape, location and in-

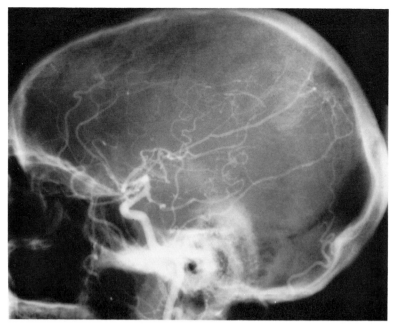

Figure 239 A. *Left lateral cerebral angiogram (arterial phase).*

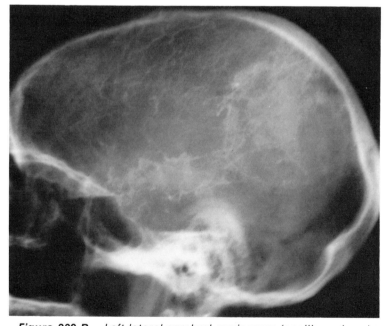

Figure 239 B. *Left lateral cerebral angiogram (capillary phase).*

tense radionuclide accumulation almost immediately following the onset of symptoms does not suggest a cerebral vascular accident. Lesions that give this appearance are arteriovenous malformations, vascular metastases, some meningiomas and Grade IV astrocytomas (glioblastoma multiforme). Arterio-venous malformations will often be seen only faintly on delayed studies. Metastases *may* be single lesions, but are usually multiple. Glioblastomas characteristically are single large, very vascular lesions. The radioactivity usually disappears at about the same rate as from other vascular structures. A cerebral angiogram (Figure 239 A and B) was obtained which shows large irregular vessels in the parietal region. There is a "tumor stain" on the capillary phase. This stain is most intense and homogeneous at the periphery of the lesion. The most probable diagnosis is glioblastoma multiforme, but one could reasonably consider a vascular meningioma.

Diagnosis: A glioblastoma multiforme was found at surgery. Often there is no characteristic location of the abnormality on the brain scan and no radiographic clue as to the diagnosis even on angiography, but the patient's clinical history makes the diagnosis seem certain.

PROBLEM

Sherwood Malthus, 21, has had a congenital heart defect since birth. Several days prior to admission the patient had an unexplained fever. He gradually became somnolent and was unconscious when seen at our hospital. His skull radiographs were normal. The brain scan was obtained (Figure 240 A and B) as well as a cerebral angiogram (Figure 241). Is there a lesion in the same location on the two studies? Does the angiogram further characterize the lesion? What is the most likely diagnosis? Do you base this upon the scan, the angiogram or the clinical history?

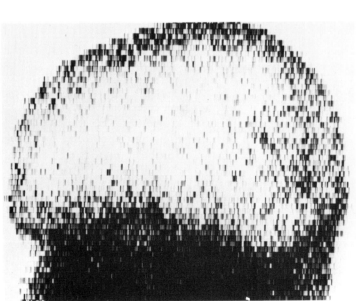

Figure 240 A. *Mr. Malthus, left lateral scan.*

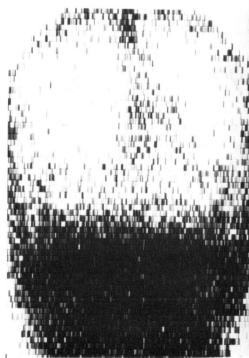

Figure 240 B. *Mr. Malthus, posterior view.*

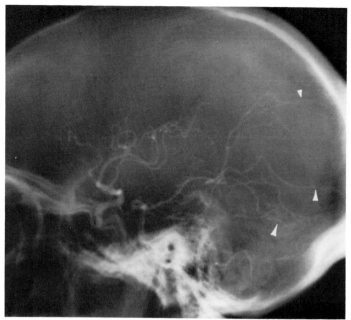

Figure 241. Sherwood Malthus, cerebral angiogram.

INTERPRETATION: The left occipital lesion on the left lateral and posterior brain scan is not further characterized by the angiogram, which only shows vessel displacement (arrows). We were as impressed with the history as you were and called this a cerebral abscess. The abscess was surgically evacuated and contrast material placed in the cavity. A follow-up lateral skull radiograph (Figure 242) shows the extent of the cavity.

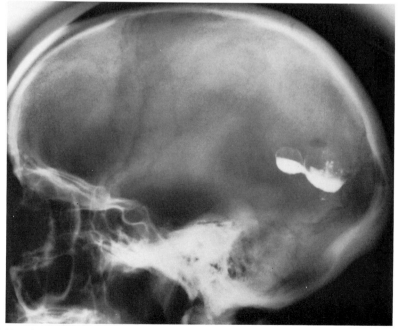

Figure 242. Lateral skull radiograph (abscess injection with sterile contrast medium).

PROBLEM

Brodie Tarkington has been chosen as our final patient for this section because he allows us to use several diagnostic modalities to arrive at a specific and, hopefully, accurate diagnosis. The patient's illness had lasted several years, during which he had changed from a pious foreman and head of a household to an irresponsible, irascible man incapable of intelligent planned activity. As part of his neurological evaluation the brain scan was obtained on the scintillation camera (Figure 243 *A*, *B* and *C*, lateral, anterior and vertex). The concomitant skull radiograph should also be analyzed (Figure 244 *A*).

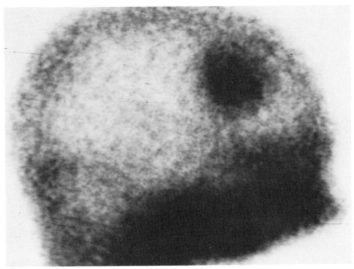

Figure 243 A. *Mr. B. Tarkington, right lateral brain scan (camera view).*

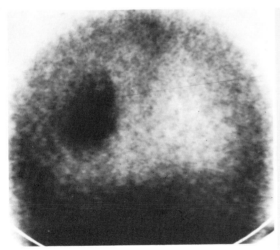

Figure 243 B. *Mr. B. T., anterior view.*

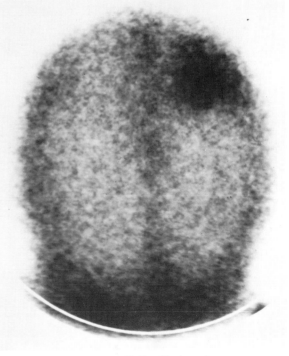

Figure 243 C. *Vertex view.*

CLUE: Particular attention should be directed to the vascular grooves on the skull radiograph. Is there any asymmetry? What common intracranial neoplasm has both an internal and external carotid blood supply?

The dynamic study was obtained in the vertex position (Figure 245 B). This is an early venous phase. How would you characterize the amount of radio-activity in the lesion compared with the superior sagittal sinus?

Summarize the long history, peripheral nature of the lesion, its external blood supply and the radionuclide accumulation; then select the most probable diagnosis.

Diagnosis: This patient had a frontal lobe meningioma.

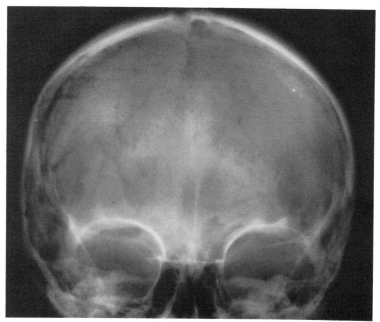

Figure 244 A. *Anteroposterior skull radiograph.*

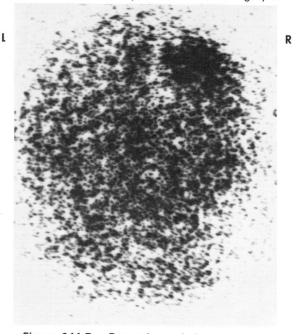

Figure 244 B. *Dynamic study (vertex view).*

CISTERNOGRAPHY

Injection of an appropriate radiopharmaceutical into the subarachnoid space to document the distribution and movement of cerebrospinal fluid has clinical utility. This study has been effectively employed (1) to evaluate and classify hydrocephalus, (2) to detect and quantify cerebrospinal fluid fistulas, (3) to determine and quantify the patency of cerebrospinal fluid diversionary shunts, and (4) to evaluate movement and absorption of cerebrospinal fluid in patients with many neurological disorders.

Hydrocephalus may generally be divided into noncommunicating (obstructive) hydrocephalus and communicating hydrocephalus. Under the broad category of communicating hydrocephalus there are two general types in which: (1) the primary process is atrophy of neural tissue, and (2) there is an obstruction to CSF flow outside of the ventricular system but within the subarachnoid space.

Radiopharmaceutical injected into the lumbar intrathecal space in patients with normal cerebrospinal fluid circulation will pass into the basal cisterns by two to six hours, and will be seen concentrated within the parasagittal region within 24 to 48 hours. With obstructive hydrocephalus, a normal pattern may be seen because there is no ventricular entry of the radiopharmaceutical normally. However, with increased intracranial pressure there may be obliteration of the basal cisterns and failure of movement of the radiopharmaceutical up over the cerebral convexities. Therefore, on the 24- and 48-hour images, the radiopharmaceutical may remain within the basal cistern area and within the subarachnoid space of the cervical spine region.

In communicating hydrocephalus entry of radiopharmaceutical into the ventricular system occurs. You can see this best in the area of the lateral ventricles since they are the largest and contain the greatest amount of radioactivity. There may be continued presence of radiopharmaceutical in the lateral ventricles on delayed images at 24 and 48 hours. The presence of radiopharmaceutical for these protracted time periods has been termed "stasis" and has been correlated with clinical improvement from cerebrospinal fluid diversionary shunts.

Other neurological diseases which affect the cerebrospinal fluid space and are reflected in abnormalities of movement of cerebrospinal fluid may be diagnosed by CSF imaging. Peripheral neoplasms, such as cerebellopontine angle tumors, may alter the configuration of the CSF space and be detected. Localized enlargement of the CSF space associated with porencephalic cysts, focal brain atrophy and congenital malformations (such as Dandy-Walker cysts) may be evaluated and diagnosed by cisternography. Not only do you demonstrate the anatomical abnormality, but its physiological and functional significance can be assessed.

Normal Cisternographic Images

The artist's drawing (Figure 245) of the distribution of the radioactivity at two hours after lumbar injection on the anterior and lateral views shows a major amount of radioactivity to be within the basal and Sylvian cisterns (shaded area). Below the drawing, the corresponding normal anterior and lateral cisternograms are seen (Figure 246 A and B). Areas containing radioactivity correspond to the shaded areas in the drawing. Figure 247 is a stylized drawing at 24 hours and shows the distribution of radioactivity denoted by the shaded areas. The radioactivity should be selectively accumulated in the parasagittal

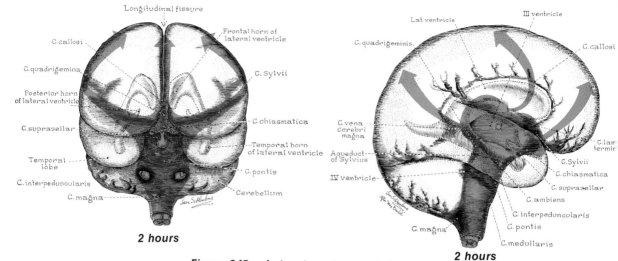

Figure 245. *A drawing of normal cisternogram.*

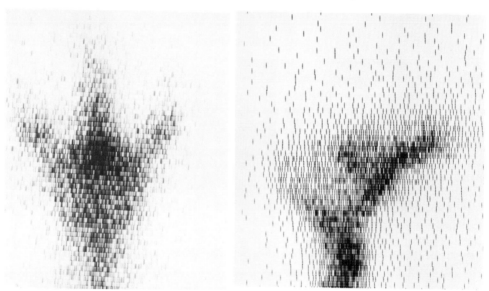

Figure 246 A. *Anterior scan.*

Figure 246 B. *Right lateral view at two hours.*

(*Figure 246 from DeLand, F. H.: Continuing Education Series, Southeastern Chapter, Soc. Nuc. Med., 1972.*)

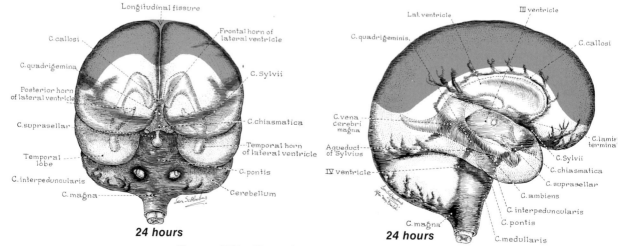

Figure 247. *Normal anterior and lateral views.*

(*Figures 245 and 247 from James, A. E., DeBlanc, H. J., Wagner, H. N., New, P. F. J., and DeLand, F. H.: Rad. Revista, 6:23–24, 1971.*)

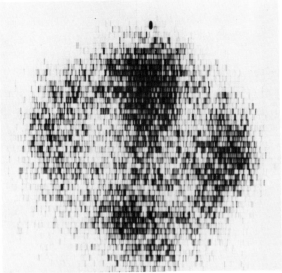

Figure 248 A. *Anterior cisternogram at 24 hours. (From James, A. E., DeBlanc, H. J., Wagner, H. N., New, P. F. J., and DeLand, F. H.: Rad. Revista, 6:23–24, 1971.)*

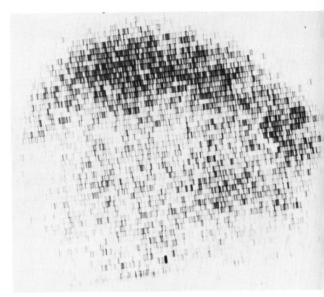

Figure 248 B. *Right lateral normal cisternogram at 24 hours.*

region by 24 hours. The normal anterior and right lateral 24 hour cisternographic views are shown (Figure 248 A and B).

Retention of the major amount of radioactivity within the basilar cisterns or entry and stasis of the radioactivity within the lateral ventricles is distinctly abnormal.

COMMUNICATING HYDROCEPHALUS

In communicating hydrocephalus, there is concentration of radioactivity within all the ventricles, but because of their size you will only see the lateral ventricles (Figure 249). On the anterior view this is a somewhat heart-shaped area of radioactivity. On the lateral view an obliquely oriented "C" is seen. The posterior view demonstrates the radioactivity within the lateral ventricles in a "butterfly" configuration. If you are not certain why the radio-pharmaceutical seems to flow "backward" into the ventricles in communicating hydrocephalus you are among the majority. Ventricular entry of the radiopharmaceutical from a lumbar sub-arachnoid injection correlates with dilatation and probably with secondary absorption of CSF in the ventricular area.

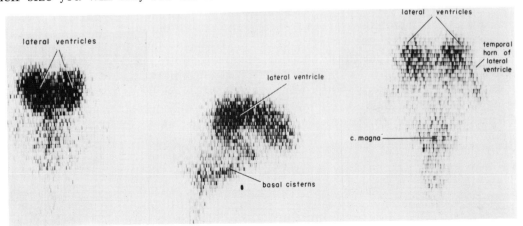

Figure 249. *Communicating hydrocephalus. (From DeLand, F. H., James, A. E., Wagner, H. N., and Hosain, F.: J. Nucl. Med., 12:683–689, 1971.)*

PROBLEM

Let's consider the plight of **Wendy Head**, 56, who several years ago had a vascular clip placed on an aneurysm. She enters now with clinical signs of hydrocephalus. The skull radiograph and six-hour anterior view of the cisternogram (Figure 250 *A* and *B*) show both the abnormality and the cause. Is there radiopharmaceutical in the ventricle? Is this radiopharmaceutical flow in the Sylvian areas symmetrical?

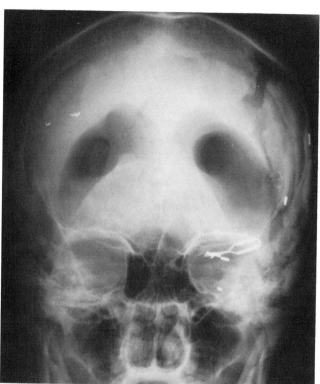

Figure 250 A. *Wendy Head, skull radiograph after pneumoencephalogram.*

Figure 250 B. *Anterior view, cisternogram. (From DeLand, F. H., James, A. E., Wagner, H. N., and Hosain, F.: J. Nucl. Med., 12:683–689, 1971.)*

INTERPRETATION: On the skull radiograph, a posteroanterior view taken after a pneumoencephalogram, air is seen within the dilated lateral ventricles and a surgical clip overlies the left orbit. In addition to the surgical clip there is evidence of a craniotomy with large drill holes joined by a linear incision into the bony calvarium itself. Surgical clips were placed on the dura.

On the anterior view of the cisternogram, you see no radioactivity flowing up the left side. However, centrally there is a "heart-shaped" configuration characteristic of radioactivity in the lateral ventricles. Therefore, ventricular enlargement is present by both modalities, pneumoencephalography and cisternography. Entry of the radiopharmaceutical into the ventricles is explained by the fact that no flow of radiopharmaceutical over the left convexity is present. You might imagine that the cerebrospinal fluid space on the left side has been obliterated by the previous surgery. This can occur after hemorrhage or trauma as a result of fibrous healing. It also happens acutely in hemorrhage or meningitis as a result of acute inflammatory reaction or filling of a peripheral CSF pathway with blood.

TEACHING POINT: The CSF, which is mainly produced in the choroid plexus of the ventricles, cannot flow up over one cerebral hemisphere to the area of greatest absorption (the arachnoid villi in the parasagittal area). Ventricular enlargement ensues and you have communicating hydrocephalus.

PROBLEM

Joseph O'Flaherty, 51, better known as "Honest Joe," a large volume used car dealer of some local repute, is evaluated for decreasing mentation. It seems that "Honest Joe" had actually been giving some honest deals and as a result had not enjoyed his usual profit margin for the past two years. On physical examination, he demonstrated minimal incoordination to fine motion and an awkwardness to purposeful movement. Pneumoencephalogram and cisternograms were obtained.

The lateral and anterior view of the 24-hour cisternograms (Figures 251 A and B) are oriented to correspond with the pneumoencephalogram (Figures 252 A and B). Are the ventricles enlarged? Does air or radiopharmaceutical get up over the cerebral cortex?

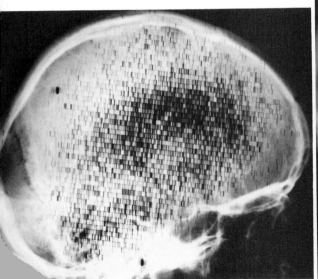
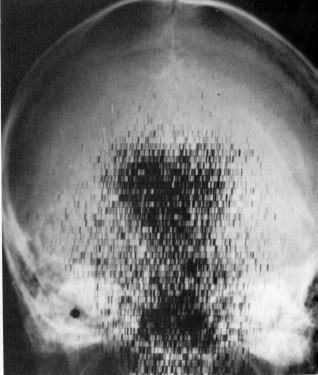

Figure 251. Honest Joe O'Flaherty lateral (A) and anterior (B) views. (From DeLand, F. H., and Wagner, H. N.: Atlas of Nuclear Medicine, Vol. 1, 1969.)

INTERPRETATION: On the pneumoencephalogram there is marked dilatation of the lateral ventricles with failure of air to flow over the cerebral convexities. The pneumoencephalographic findings are again physiologically demonstrated by the cisternogram. The lateral and anterior view show radioactivity within the lateral ventricles and no movement of radioactivity to the parasagittal region, which is characteristic of a certain form of communicating hydrocephalus. Because of the stasis of the radiopharmaceutical, the patient's history, pneumoencephalogram, and findings at lumbar puncture, the partic-

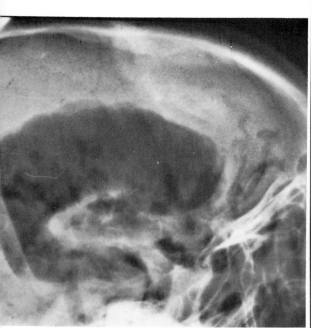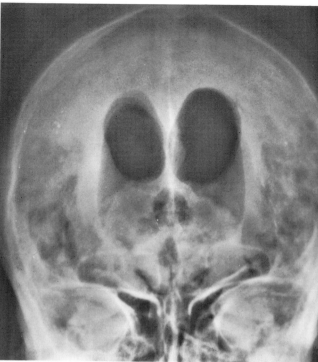

Figure 252. *Lateral* (A) *and posterior* (B) *views of pneumoencephalogram. (From James, A. E., DeLand, F. H., Hodges, F. J., and Wagner, H. N.: J.A.M.A., 213:1615, 1970.)*

ular syndrome is termed "normal pressure" hydrocephalus. It may be just a form of communicating hydrocephalus in which the obliteration of the cerebrospinal fluid space is in the parasagittal region, or it may be that obstruction to CSF flow is physiological rather than mechanical. You have probably encountered this entity in the recent literature as there has been great interest in identifying these patients because they respond to CSF diversionary shunts.

Diagnosis: Normal pressure hydrocephalus.

TEACHING POINT: In the syndrome of "normal pressure" hydrocephalus, there is marked enlargement of the ventricles. The ventricular entry of the radiopharmaceutical is great and it remains there for protracted time periods (stasis). There is markedly diminished flow to the parasagittal region. These findings may explain why removal of the CSF from the ventricular area by a diversionary shunt into the peritoneum or venous system results in dramatic neurological improvement.

PROBLEM

Countess Hermione von Goetrocks, 39, going on 63, enters with a four-year history of diffuse disorientation, forgetfulness and diminished reasoning ability. Pneumoencephalogram (Figure 253 A) and cisternogram (Figure 253 B and C, anterior and lateral, six-hour) were obtained to evaluate the patient for the possibility of "normal pressure" hydrocephalus. A delayed lateral cisternographic view was also made (Figure 253 D).

Compare the pneumoencephalogram (PEG) (Figure 253 A) with that of Honest Joe O'Flaherty (Figure 252 B). Are the ventricles as large and were we able to get air over the Countess' cerebral cortex (Figure 253 A)? The two lateral views of the cisternogram were at six and 48 hours after injection. Does the radiopharmaceutical flow up over the cerebral cortex by 48 hours? Are the findings similar to but somewhat different from the previous case?

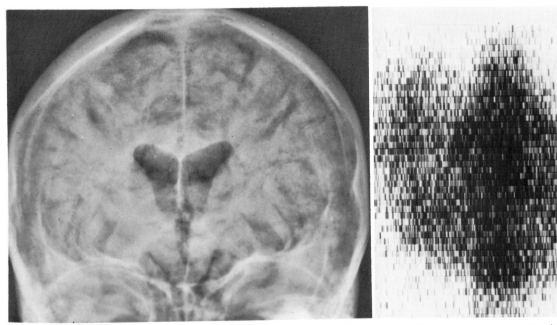

Figure 253 A. *Pneumoencephalogram.*   **Figure 253 B.** *Anterior scan at six hours.*

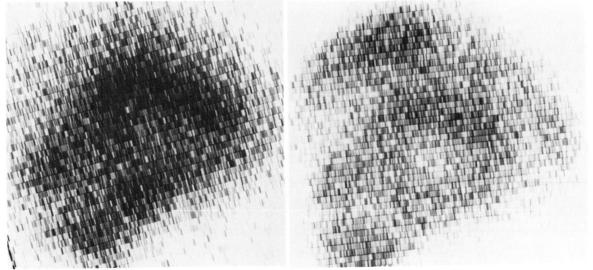

Figure 253 C. *Right lateral scan at six hours.*   **Figure 253 D.** *Right lateral scan at 48 hours.*

(Figure 253 B & C from DeLand, F. H., and Wagner, H. N.: Atlas of Nuclear Medicine, Vol. 1, 1969.)

INTERPRETATION: On the anterior view of the pneumoencephalogram and corresponding anterior cisternogram, air and radiopharmaceutical are seen within minimally enlarged ventricles. Air is distributed over the cerebral convexity. Dilated sulci are visualized.

On the six-hour anterior cisternogram you see radioactivity centrally within the lateral ventricles. On the lateral view at six hours, there is radioactivity in the lateral ventricles as well as some over the cerebral cortex. By 48 hours radioactivity has concentrated in the parasagittal region and there has been movement of radioactivity up over the cerebral cortex. Minimal radioactivity, however, remains within the lateral ventricles. From the pneumoencephalogram and the distribution of radioactivity over the time period seen on the cisternogram, this patient has communicating hydrocephalus. However, this is of the type seen in primary brain atrophy.

Diagnosis: Communicating hydroceph-alus due to generalized brain atrophy.

TEACHING POINT: This is communicating hydrocephalus because the radiopharmaceutical goes into the ventricles. However, it also gets up over the cortex and concentrates in the parasagittal region by 48 hours. Thus, the pattern is entry *without stasis*, the most common cause of which is generalized atrophy.

PROBLEM
Oliver Widegate, 47, is evaluated because of ataxia and incoordination. A cisternogram (Figure 254) and PEG (Figure 255 *A* and *B*) were obtained to evaluate the possibility of "normal pressure" hydrocephalus or a posterior fossa lesion. The posterior view of the cisternogram at 24 hours is shown with an upright posteroanterior and lateral view of the PEG designed to visualize the posterior fossa structures. Is there any localized area in which radiopharmaceutical is abnormally accumulated?

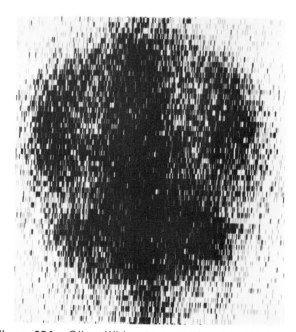

Figure 254. Oliver Widegate, posterior view (24 hours).

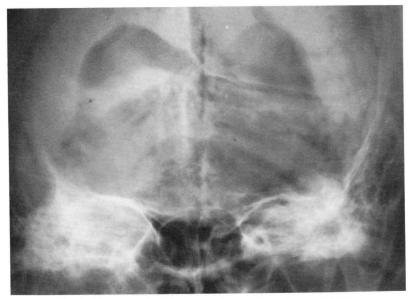

Figure 255 A. *Posterior fossa view, pneumoencephalogram.*

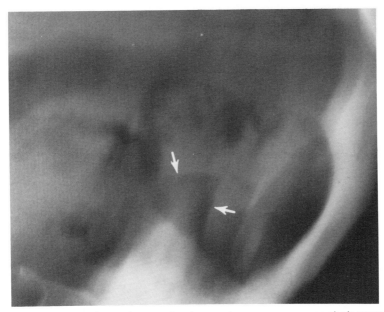

Figure 255 B. *Lateral posterior fossa view, pneumoencephalogram.*

INTERPRETATION: On the 24-hour posterior view of the cisternogram, concentration of radioactivity in the posterior basal region is present. This appears to be within the cerebellar area. Concentration of radioactivity within this area *may* be seen as a normal variant. However, concentration of radioactivity to this extent on the 24-hour study is distinctly unusual.

The pneumoencephalogram on the anterior and left lateral views shows dilatation of the space around the cerebellar folia (streaky transverse collections of air), as well as a small cerebellum and enlargement of the fourth ventricle. The fourth ventricle (arrows) is noted as the triangular structure in the midportion of the cerebellum. These radiographic signs as well as the cisternogram are characteristic of cerebellar atrophy.

PROBLEM

Owen Evenfors, 56, has had a cerebrospinal fluid diversionary shunt because of a fourth ventricular ependymoma and subsequent noncommunicating hydrocephalus. A cisternogram was performed from a lumbar injection to determine if, with the shunt, there was flow of the cerebrospinal fluid up over the cerebral convexities to the parasagittal region (Figure 256 A and B). These views are obtained 24 hours after lumbar injection (superimposed on the skull radiograph for your orientation). Do you think that normal progression to the parasagittal region has occurred?

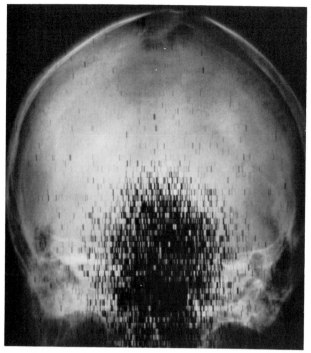

Figure 256 A. *Owen Evenfors, anterior view.*

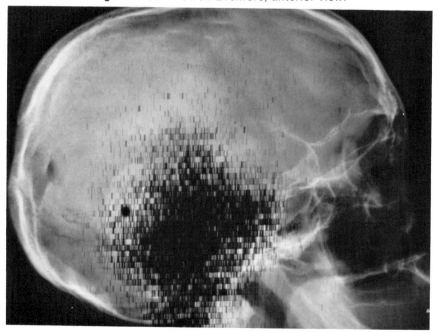

Figure 256 B. *Owen Evenfors, right lateral view.*
(*Figure 256 A & B from DeLand, F. H., and Wagner, H. N.:* Atlas of Nuclear Medicine, *Vol. 1, 1969.*)

ANSWER: At 24 hours on the anterior and right lateral cisternograms, radioactivity remains concentrated within the basal cisterns. This appearance is seen in patients with noncommunicating forms of hydrocephalus and is felt to be due to increased intracranial pressure. No ventricular entry occurred and there has been no concentration of radioactivity in the parasagittal region by 24 hours.

CEREBROSPINAL FLUID DIVERSIONARY SHUNT EVALUATION

PROBLEM
Henry Bridges, 43, has had a ventriculoperitoneal cerebrospinal fluid diversionary shunt (Figure 257) following subacute meningitis and a basilar arachnoiditis. A cisternogram was obtained (Figure 258). There is a partial communication to cerebrospinal fluid flow as radioactivity is seen in the subarachnoid space of the thoracic and lumbar spine. *Henry* does have some communication between the basal cisterns and the ventricles. The lateral ventricle was injected with the radiopharmaceutical through the shunt (Figure 258). This is seen as the most superior image in an anterior view on the composite (*A*). Below this is an image of the radioactivity within the spinal canal (*B*). The paired structures on each side of the spinal radioactivity represent what organs?

CLUE: This is a chelated radiopharmaceutical and is eliminated from the body by glomerular filtration. If you have figured out what the paired structures are, then you might attempt the lowest image. You see a spherical area of radioactivity with a very dense linear band of radioactivity leading from it (*C*).

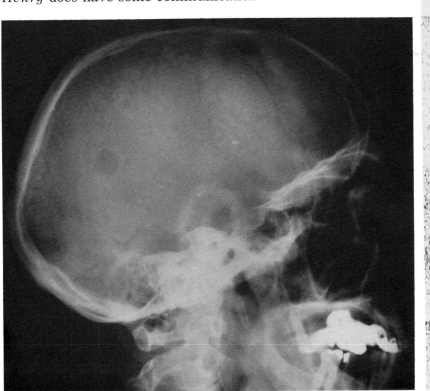

Figure 257. *Henry Bridges, right lateral skull radiograph.* **Figure 258.** *Mr. Bridges.*
(Figure 258 from DeLand, F. H., James, A. E., Wagner, H. N., and Hosain, F.: J. Nucl. Med., *12:683, 1971.)*

ANSWER: Doubtless you have already concluded that the paired areas of radioactivity are the kidneys. The rounded area of radioactivity in the image below is the urinary bladder. What you were not expected to figure out was that the linear area of radioactivity is a suprapubic catheter.

This study shows that there is communication between the ventricles and the lumbar subarachnoid space. It also demonstrates by the presence of radioactivity in the intraperitoneal space that the ventriculoperitoneal shunt is functioning. The radioactivity within the urinary system present in the first two hours of the study further demonstrates in a physiological manner the patency of the shunt.

Diagnosis: CSF diversionary shunt, patent.

PROBLEM

James E. Brown, 8, has a posterior fossa neoplasm and obstructive hydrocephalus due to obliteration of the fourth ventricle and obstruction of the aqueduct of Sylvius. A CSF diversionary shunt has been placed into the markedly enlarged lateral ventricle (Figure 259 A). The distal tip lies intraperitonally just below the left hemidiaphragm.

Injection of the radiopharmaceutical within the proximal portion of the shunt is seen on the anterior view since both the shunt (arrow) and lateral ventricle (triangle) activity are noted (Figure 259 B). On the lower part of the image at two hours, there is a linear band of radioactivity within the lumbar region showing that the noncommunicating aspect of the hydrocephalus is not complete. What does the image over the 12th rib tell you?

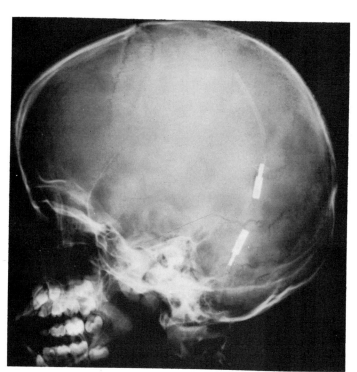

Figure 259 A. *James Brown, left lateral skull radiograph.*

(Figure 259 B from James, A. E., Hurley, P. J., Heller, R. M., and Freeman, J. M.: Annales Radiologie, *14:598, 1971.)*

Figure 259 B.

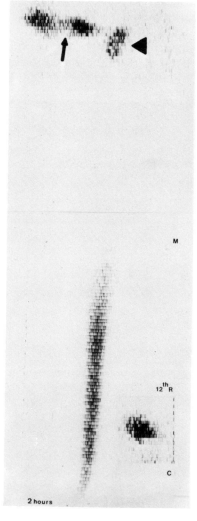

2 hours

INTERPRETATION: There is radioactivity seen over the distal shunt tip which demonstrates the patency of the CSF diversionary shunt.

Diagnosis: Patent CSF diversionary shunt.

EVALUATION OF CEREBROSPINAL FLUID FISTULAS

From a lumbar injection, images can be obtained to detect radioactivity outside the normal confines of the cerebrospinal fluid space.

PROBLEM

Martin Heigh, 8, is evaluated postsurgically for the possibility of a cerebrospinal fluid fistula. This left lateral skull radiograph (Figure 260) and seven-hour lateral cisternographic image (Figure 261) were obtained. Could you give a differential for the bizarre configuration of the skull? Is there any unexpected extension of radioactivity?

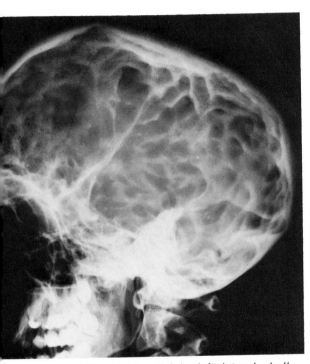

Figure 260. *Martin Heigh, left lateral skull radiograph.*

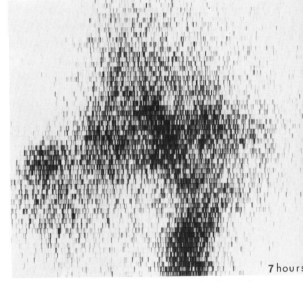

Figure 261. *Martin Heigh, left lateral cisternogram.*

(Figures 260 and 261 from James, A. E., Hurley, P. J., Heller, R. M., and Freeman, J. M.: Annales Radiologie, 14:598, 1971.)

INTERPRETATION: The left lateral skull film shows increased convolutional markings, with a distinctly abnormal skull shape in which the frontal region is particularly prominent and the floor of the anterior cranial fossa runs obliquely upward. This patient had characteristic facial features as well as the radiographic signs of Cruzon's syndrome.

The seven-hour left lateral cisternogram shows abnormal radioactivity within the frontal region, giving the so-called "Snoopy scan" appearance of a CSF fistula (Figure 261).

Diagnosis: Cerebrospinal fluid fistula through the cribriform plate into the nasal area secondary to surgery.

CONCLUSION

In this book we have illustrated a number of the basic principles of nuclear imaging. By discussion and selection of some of the examples shown, both the virtues and limitations of the specialty have been illustrated. The ability to utilize minute amounts of radiation to trace the normal and altered physiological functions of the body is a most important advance which nuclear medicine offers to the effective practice of medicine. That this leads to easy quantification of body areas and sub-areas as well as to an over-all assessment of function for comparison with normals is an exciting new diagnostic approach to disease. Comparison with other abnormalities and sequential comparison in the same patient add a dynamic continuity, with many as yet unrealized research possibilities.

Probably the greatest limitation of nuclear medicine procedures at present is the less than precise structural information contained in the images. When you compare images made with radiopharmaceuticals with those of plain radiography and contrast angiography, you can see at once that there exists a difference of great magnitude in the accurate portrayal of anatomical detail. We can only say that, although the present images are certainly not optimal, they represent a great improvement over those that were found useful clinically just a few years ago.

The development of radiopharmaceuticals that are short-lived, that are of appropriate energy, and that are pure gamma emitters, coupled with the development of large field stationary imaging devices with good spatial and temporal resolution, has greatly improved the utility of these diagnostic studies. Innovations of data storage and analysis allow even greater extraction of clinically useful information.

The constant stimulus of demands made by men in related clinical branches of medicine *is* leading to the continued development of improved imaging devices and better radiopharmaceuticals; and we can anticipate future improvement in the structural information present on nuclear medicine images. The physiological information contained in these studies has been extremely useful, not only in patient care but in giving us insight into the proper interpretation of *radiographic* images. The correlation of plain radiographs and contrast angiograms with nuclear medicine studies, as emphasized in this book, has led to greatly improved patient treatment. The use of non-invasive techniques to replace time-consuming, hazardous, and expensive studies will continue to improve the delivery of health care.

Another important and useful aspect of nuclear medicine—in vitro studies without concomitant images—we have not discussed because it is not subject to illustration. We are certain that our reading audience is aware of these studies and will seek the proper texts where they are described in detail. We also would be remiss if we failed to mention the diagnostic modality of ultrasound. In the future, this may well be the non-invasive method of choice to delineate anatomy. We can anticipate already that in many clinical circumstances ultrasound will be used to determine structural detail and trace amounts of radioactive material will be employed to obtain physiological data.

Increased utilization of scientific advances developed in other disciplines is one of the most exciting aspects of the radiologic profession as we approach the last quarter of the twentieth century. This is especially true for sub-specialty nuclear radiology. If this book has created in the reader an interest in learning more about the field and about the employment of some of these studies in the care of patients, the undertaking has been a success.

INDEX

(NOTE: This is not really a formal index at all! Rather, it is simply meant to help you find something you want to see over again. Page numbers in **boldface** refer to page on which illustration may be found; those in lightface refer to discussion in the text.)